STUDY GUIDE TO
CHILD AND ADOLESCENT
PSYCHIATRY

A Companion to
The American Psychiatric Publishing
Textbook of Child and Adolescent Psychiatry,
Third Edition

STUDY GUIDE TO CHILD AND ADOLESCENT PSYCHIATRY

A Companion to
The American Psychiatric Publishing
Textbook of Child and Adolescent Psychiatry,
Third Edition

Stephen J. Cozza, M.D.

Colonel, U.S. Army Medical Corps
Chief, Department of Psychiatry, Walter Reed Army Medical Center
Washington, D.C.
Associate Professor of Psychiatry and Associate Director, Center for the Study of Traumatic Stress,
Uniformed Services University of the Health Sciences
Bethesda, Maryland

Robert E. Hales, M.D., M.B.A.

Joe P. Tupin Professor and Chair, Department of Psychiatry and Behavioral Sciences
University of California–Davis School of Medicine
Director, UC Davis Health System Behavioral Health Center
Director, UC Davis Sierra Health Foundation MD/MBA Fellowship Program
Medical Director, Mental Health Services, County of Sacramento
Sacramento, California

Narriman C. Shahrokh

Chief Administrative Officer, Department of Psychiatry and Behavioral Sciences
University of California–Davis School of Medicine
Sacramento, California

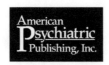

American Psychiatric Publishing, Inc.
Washington, DC
London, England

Copyright © 2006 American Psychiatric Publishing, Inc.

ALL RIGHTS RESERVED

Manufactured in the United States of America on acid-free paper
10   09   08   07   06   5   4   3   2   1

ISBN   1-58562-261-3
ISBN-13   978-1-58562-261-0

First Edition

Typeset in Revival BT and Adobe's The Mix

American Psychiatric Publishing, Inc.
1000 Wilson Boulevard
Arlington, VA 22209-3901
www.appi.org

Contents

Answer Guide

Page numbers in the Answer Guide refer to *The American Psychiatric Publishing Textbook of Child and Adolescent Psychiatry,* Third Edition. Visit **www.appi.org** for more information about this textbook.

| | | |

Purchase the online version of this Study Guide at

www.cme.psychiatryonline.org

and receive instant scoring and CME credits.

C H A P T E R   1

Development of the Subspecialty of Child and Adolescent Psychiatry in the United States

Select the single best response for each question.

1.1   The initial purposes of the Academy of Child Psychiatry included all of the following *except*

 A. Delineate the scope of the specialty and its practice.
 B. Set standards of training and practice.
 C. Stimulate physicians to enter the field of child psychiatry.
 D. Enroll all practicing child psychiatrists.
 E. Promote and advance prevention, treatment, research, and teaching in the field.

1.2   Erik Erikson's classic text *Childhood and Society* (1950) emphasized the principles of which of the following as important for understanding normal development and psychopathology in childhood?

 A. Psychoanalysis.
 B. Ego psychology.
 C. Family therapy.
 D. Behavior therapy.
 E. Crisis intervention.

1.3   Szurek (1942) and Johnson (1949) used the term *superego lacunae* to describe which of the following?

 A. Neuronal abnormalities in cortical development of delinquents.
 B. Gaps in family structure (parental absence) in the families of delinquent adolescents.
 C. Positive magnetic resonance imaging findings suggesting basal ganglia pathology in delinquents.
 D. Developmental abnormalities in the language functioning of delinquents.
 E. The contribution of unconscious parental permission to the antisocial acts of delinquents.

1.4   Which of the following researchers focused on the important contributions of temperament to child development?

 A. Chess and Thomas.
 B. Bowlby.
 C. Piaget.
 D. Spitz.
 E. Brazelton.

1.5   Which of the following statements about managed care and its impact on child psychiatry is *false*?

A. Managed care was designed to contain the rising costs of health care.
B. Managed care may limit the ability of child psychiatrists to provide adequate care to patients.
C. Managed care decisions related to treatments of choice are based on well-documented and well-conducted outcome studies.
D. Managed care may require child psychiatrists to serve in an advocacy role for their patients.
E. Managed care decisions may be driven more by cost considerations than by treatment considerations.

CHAPTER 2

Overview of Development From Infancy Through Adolescence

Select the single best response for each question.

2.1 Theories of development formulated by Freud, Erikson, and Piaget share which of the following characteristics?

A. They postulate a genetically determined capacity for the development of patterns or systems of behavior by the child.
B. They propose that the overall behavior patterns that emerge are qualitatively similar to one another.
C. They are all structural theories of development that imply that reorganization within the child is unnecessary.
D. They postulate that the child reacts in particular ways to environmental stimuli.
E. None of the above.

2.2 By age 5 years, a child will have attained all of the following motor developmental milestones *except*

A. Can stand on one foot.
B. Can dance and jump.
C. Manifests firmly established leg, eye, and ear dominance.
D. Can copy a square.
E. Can build a tower of 10 cubes.

2.3 Piaget conceptualized four major stages of cognitive development. Which of the following states the correct sequence in which these stages normally occur, from birth to adolescence?

A. Preoperational, sensorimotor, concrete operational, formal operational.
B. Concrete operational, sensorimotor, preoperational, formal operational.
C. Sensorimotor, concrete operational, formal operational, preoperational.
D. Formal operational, concrete operational, sensorimotor, preoperational.
E. Sensorimotor, preoperational, concrete operational, formal operational.

2.4   Chunking is

   A. A process by which representations, procedures, and memories that occur together are
       automatically accessed simultaneously.
   B. A type of long-term memory.
   C. A form of procedural knowledge.
   D. All of the above.
   E. None of the above.

2.5   According to Spitz (1965), organizers that govern the process of transition from one level to the next
       in the development of attachment include all of the following *except*

   A. Sustained eye contact in response to an interaction.
   B. The smiling response.
   C. Eight-month anxiety.
   D. Achievement of the sign of negation.
   E. None of the above.

2.6   In psychoanalytic theory, the *anal phase* of psychosexual development is characterized by

   A. The child's focus on autoerotic activities.
   B. The child's experience of intense sexual and aggressive urges toward both parents.
   C. The child's development of concepts of inevitability regarding birth, death, and sex differences.
   D. The child's experience of feelings of separateness and worth.
   E. The child's sequential development of play.

C H A P T E R   3

Role of Culture, Race, and Ethnicity in Child and Adolescent Psychiatry

Select the single best response for each question.

3.1   Terms such as *race*, *ethnicity*, *culture*, and *nationality* are often used synonymously, but each represents a distinct concept. For example, in North America, the term *African American* represents which of the following?

   A. Race and ethnicity.
   B. Race and culture.
   C. Ethnicity and nationality.
   D. Nationality and culture.
   E. None of the above.

3.2   Cross-cultural psychiatry

   A. Discounts the presence of culture-specific syndromes.
   B. Minimizes the universal applicability of psychiatric diagnoses.
   C. Recognizes that psychiatric conditions may have different characteristics in different cultural and ethnic groups.
   D. Emphasizes the importance of cultural over individual contributions to illness.
   E. Has little clinical research that supports its basic tenets.

3.3   Konner (1995) described five cross-cultural factors universally present in human development. Which of the following lists the correct developmental order of these factors?

   A. Emergence of socialization, onset of attachments, emergence of language, observable gender-specific aggression, mature sexual motivation.
   B. Onset of attachments, emergence of socialization, observable gender-specific aggression, emergence of language, mature sexual motivation.
   C. Onset of attachments, emergence of language, emergence of socialization, observable gender-specific aggression, mature sexual motivation.
   D. Emergence of language, onset of attachments, emergence of socialization, observable gender-specific aggression, mature sexual motivation.
   E. Emergence of socialization, onset of attachments, observable gender-specific aggression, emergence of language, mature sexual motivation.

3.4   Cultural assimilation

A. Refers to acquiring the norms and values of one's own cultural group.
B. Is equivalent to biculturalism.
C. Represents the desire to replace one's own cultural values with those of the host culture.
D. Allows one to retain significant portions of one's own cultural values while absorbing those of another.
E. Is correlated with a lower risk of psychopathology in Hispanic adolescents.

3.5   All of the following statements about the African American cultural experience in the United States are correct *except*

A. African Americans constitute the largest minority group in the United States.
B. African Americans experience higher levels of social, emotional, and financial distress than do whites, regardless of socioeconomic status.
C. Extended kinship networks provide emotional support for many African American families.
D. Religious belief and church affiliation provide support to many African Americans.
E. Stereotypic impressions of African Americans can result in ineffective treatment.

C H A P T E R   4

Economic Issues in Child and Adolescent Psychiatry

Select the single best response for each question.

4.1   Which of the following is a strategy used by managed care organizations (MCOs) to contain costs for mental health services?

   A. Placing gatekeepers between patients and mental health providers.
   B. Requiring precertification.
   C. Channeling patients to the least expensive providers.
   D. Using prospective payment plans.
   E. All of the above.

4.2   Which of the following is an anticipated outcome of a single-payer health care financing model?

   A. Risk would be spread over a smaller segment of the population.
   B. Administrative overhead would most certainly increase.
   C. Payment for health care would shift from premium dollars to tax dollars.
   D. Uninsured people would be excluded from care.
   E. None of the above.

4.3   In the defined-contribution health plan arrangement, the employer

   A. Selects one health insurance plan for all employees.
   B. Carries over payments not used by employees to the next year.
   C. Provides a tax-sheltered account that may not be carried over to the next year.
   D. Caps the contribution it is willing to make.
   E. Remains the payer.

4.4   Disease management systems aim to promote wellness by managing risk in patients and in the population so as to improve outcomes in quality and cost of health care. Strategies employed to meet these goals include all of the following *except*

   A. Early detection of vulnerable individuals.
   B. Reliance on individual physician practice decisions.
   C. Patient education to empower self-management.
   D. Process and outcomes measurement, evaluation, and management.
   E. Use of a routine reporting/feedback loop.

4.5   According to Epidemiologic Catchment Area (ECA) study estimations, what percentage of Americans (including children and adolescents) in any given year had a diagnosable psychiatric disorder that required treatment?

   A. 5%.
   B. 10%.
   C. 15%.
   D. 20%.
   E. 25%.

C H A P T E R   5

Classification of Child and Adolescent Psychiatric Disorders

Select the single best response for each question.

5.1   A number of changes were made in DSM-IV (American Psychiatric Association 1994) that apply to childhood. Which of the following is one of these changes?

A. A new category of pervasive developmental disorders was to be coded on Axis II.
B. Motor skills disorders were moved from Axis II to Axis I.
C. Learning disorders were moved from Axis I to Axis II.
D. Communications disorders were moved from Axis I to Axis II.
E. None of the above.

5.2   Pervasive developmental disorders include all of the following *except*

A. Childhood schizophrenia.
B. Autistic disorder.
C. Rett's disorder.
D. Asperger's disorder.
E. Childhood disintegrative disorder.

5.3   In DSM-IV, the new category *feeding and eating disorders of infancy or early childhood* included all of the following *except*

A. Feeding disorder of infancy or early childhood (persistent failure to eat adequately, with weight loss or failure to gain weight).
B. Pica.
C. Anorexia nervosa.
D. Rumination disorder.
E. None of the above.

5.4   The tic disorders category of DSM-IV was left essentially unchanged from that in DSM-III-R (American Psychiatric Association 1987) except for which of the following?

A. The addition of Tourette's disorder.
B. The elimination of chronic motor or vocal tic disorder.
C. The lowering of the upper limit of age at onset to 18 years.
D. The addition of transient tic disorder.
E. None of the above.

5.5 In DSM-IV, the category *other disorders of infancy, childhood, or adolescence* was reorganized to include which of the following disorders?

   A. Separation anxiety disorder.
   B. Selective mutism.
   C. Reactive attachment disorder of infancy or early childhood.
   D. Stereotypic movement disorder.
   E. All of the above.

C H A P T E R   6

Concepts of Diagnostic Classification

Select the single best response for each question.

6.1   Knowledge of the diagnosis should allow the professional to make inferences about which of the following?

    A. Likely etiology of the disorder.
    B. Probable natural history of the disorder.
    C. Expected response of the disorder to specified types of treatment.
    D. The nature of other clinical conditions that are commonly associated with the disorder.
    E. All of the above.

6.2   Comorbidity between different diagnoses can arise for several reasons. Which of the following statements concerning potential causes of diagnostic comorbidity is *incorrect*?

    A. Comorbidity can arise as a result of purely structural factors, such as the presence of similar criteria in different disorders.
    B. Comorbidity can arise when two disorders lack an etiological relationship.
    C. Comorbidity can arise because the presence of one disorder has led to another as a complication.
    D. Comorbidity can arise because two disorders have common environmental or biological antecedents.
    E. All of the above.

6.3   DSM-IV-TR (American Psychiatric Association 2000) is an example of a categorical diagnostic system, in which a disorder is deemed either present or absent on the basis of whether an individual meets or does not meet certain criteria. Which of the following is an advantage of categorical diagnoses?

    A. Disorders do not always present themselves in as complete a form as are represented by the diagnostic definitions.
    B. Diagnostic criteria differ in their potential for causing impairment.
    C. The number and type of symptoms will commonly vary with the age and sex of the patient.
    D. The categorization of a disorder as being either present or absent represents the way that clinicians and patients think of disorders.
    E. All of the above.

6.4   Which of the following is a disadvantage of dimensional/empirical diagnostic systems?

A. The items in the inventories are usually written in a complicated fashion with many qualifiers.
B. Factor structure remains constant across different age and gender groups.
C. Being a "case" becomes a function of deviation from normal scores rather than of impairment that interferes with functioning.
D. The information is usually collected from multiple instruments.
E. All of the above.

6.5   Because psychosocial circumstances and stressors may affect the diagnosis, treatment, and prognosis of psychiatric disorders, documenting the presence, history, and severity of such problems is important. It may, however, be difficult for patients to accurately recall the order of stressors and behavioral or emotional problems, because

A. Most childhood disorders are chronic.
B. The influence of subclinical premorbid states on an individual's functioning is difficult to reconstruct.
C. Many childhood stressors are chronic.
D. Distortions occur as part of a search for meaning.
E. All of the above.

C H A P T E R 7

Clinical Assessment in Infancy and Early Childhood

Select the single best response for each question.

7.1   Psychiatric clinical assessment in infancy

    A. Requires a less comprehensive approach than does assessment during childhood.
    B. Should focus most extensively on cognitive development.
    C. Requires evaluation of multiple lines of development.
    D. May exclude evaluation of risk factors.
    E. Is usually best conducted after the infant reaches 6 months of age.

7.2   Which of the following prenatal and perinatal variables should be assessed in infancy?

    A. Rubella.
    B. Maternal drug or alcohol use.
    C. Complications during pregnancy or delivery.
    D. Poor maternal nutrition.
    E. All of the above.

7.3   The stage-specific task of *representational capacity, differentiation, and consolidation* (the use of ideas to guide language, pretend play, and behavior) is mastered at which of the following ages?

    A. 0–3 months.
    B. 2–7 months.
    C. 3–10 months.
    D. 9–24 months.
    E. 1.5–4 years.

7.4   The developmental, individual-difference, relationship-based (DIR) model facilitates the process of clinical assessment in infancy and early childhood by identifying, systematizing, and integrating children's essential developmental capacities. These essential capacities include all of the following *except*

    A. The child's functional–emotional developmental level.
    B. The child's academic potential.
    C. The child's individual differences in sensory–affective processing.
    D. The child's relationships and interactions with caregivers and others.
    E. The child's individual differences in motor planning and sequencing.

7.5   By the age of 12 months, a child would demonstrate all of the following capacities *except*

    A. Plays on own in a focused, organized manner for 15–20 minutes.
    B. Points and vocalizes at desired toy or object.
    C. Feeds self small finger foods.
    D. Throws a ball forward.
    E. Understands simple words or commands.

C H A P T E R   8

The Clinical Interview of the Child

Select the single best response for each question.

8.1 The Mental Health Assessment Form (MHAF)

A. May be used with children between the ages of 3 and 6 years.
B. Usually requires about 3 hours to complete.
C. Employs questionnaires.
D. Consists of 54 items.
E. Obtains information on all areas of a child's life and functioning.

8.2 The MHAF consists of two parts. Part II ("Content of the Interview") deals with all of the following areas *except*

A. Motoric behavior and speech.
B. Interpersonal relations.
C. Self-concept.
D. Feeling states.
E. Symbolic representation.

8.3 When interviewing the younger child (ages 5–9 years), the examiner should do all of the following *except*

A. Interview one or both parents before meeting the child.
B. Allow the child to examine the environment.
C. Explain the nature of the interview to the parents.
D. Refrain from explaining the reason for the interview to the child, because such information may be upsetting.
E. Provide reassurance if necessary.

8.4 When interviewing the older child (ages 10–12 years), the examiner should

A. Begin with general questions to avoid having a child get defensive about the chief complaint.
B. Start by using the MHAF designed for older children.
C. Obtain some idea about the child's development of empathy.
D. End with the chief complaint.
E. Refrain from having a parents-only meeting after the initial interview so that the child will not feel excluded.

8.5   The MHAF semistructured interview can be used to accomplish all of the following *except*

    A. Assess for the signs and symptoms of a psychiatric disorder.
    B. Identify positive attributes of the patient.
    C. Conduct a formal assessment of the patient's cognitive functioning.
    D. Establish a relationship with the patient.
    E. Evaluate the strengths of the patient.

CHAPTER 9

The Clinical Interview of the Adolescent

Select the single best response for each question.

9.1   Which of the following statements concerning the initial interview of an adolescent is *false?*

   A. Seeing the adolescent first highlights the patient's active participation in the process.
   B. Seeing the adolescent first may allay fears that the parents and therapist will gang up on the patient.
   C. The therapeutic alliance between the clinician and adolescent may be harmed if the clinician meets alone with the parents; such an approach is therefore discouraged.
   D. The clinician should make clear to the adolescent that he or she is not out to assign blame.
   E. None of the above.

9.2   Characteristic adolescent patterns of responding to interviews with a therapist include which of the following?

   A. Anxiety about revealing problems that they may regard as weaknesses.
   B. Externalization of one side or another of conflicted feelings.
   C. Counterphobic measures to deal with painful affects.
   D. An unrealistic faith in the "omnipotence of thought."
   E. All of the above.

9.3   To interview an adolescent effectively, which of the following are important qualities for a clinician?

   A. Having experienced similar problems in adolescence.
   B. Possessing a sense of humor.
   C. Being informal and familiar.
   D. Being close in age to the adolescent so that he or she can identify with the clinician.
   E. All of the above.

9.4   When should a formal mental status examination be conducted with an adolescent?

   A. When there is a concern about psychosis.
   B. When the disorder may be severe.
   C. When precise documentation is required.
   D. When there is a possibility of dementia.
   E. All of the above.

9.5   In interviewing adolescents, the therapist should

   A. Limit the interview to areas of difficulty.
   B. Demonstrate his or her familiarity with any topic that the adolescent may bring up, such as rock groups.
   C. Make early interpretations to assist the adolescent with the session.
   D. Avoid asking about dating or sexual relationships.
   E. Ask about friends and peers.

CHAPTER 10

The Parent Interview

Select the single best response for each question.

10.1 Mednick and Shaffer (1963) found that when maternal interviews were compared with pediatric records, the mothers' reports were discrepant what percentage of the time?

A. 0–6%.
B. 7%–15%.
C. 16%–20%.
D. 21%–62%.
E. 63%–75%.

10.2 A number of investigators have studied the parent interview. Which of the following descriptions of their findings is *incorrect*?

A. Weissman et al. (1987) found that parents reported far more information about their children's disorders than did the children themselves.
B. Orvaschel et al. (1981) found that parents were more accurate in providing factual time-related information.
C. Edelbrock et al. (1985) found that the reliability of a child's report increased with the child's age.
D. Edelbrock et al. (1985) found that in children 10 years of age and older, parent and child reports showed little or no difference in reliability.
E. None of the above.

10.3 Which of the following is a function of the parent interview?

A. Gathering information about the child's history.
B. Assessing the child's present functioning.
C. Identifying the child's strengths and weaknesses.
D. Giving parents information about normal child development.
E. All of the above.

10.4 The parent interview may be divided into five phases: preliminaries, prologue, interview proper, closing, and epilogue. What is the primary purpose of the *closing* phase?

A. Assess the parents' and the clinician's expectations for the interview.
B. Establish an alliance or empathetic relationship with the parents while collecting data and making the appropriate interventions.
C. Reassure the parents and reinforce their control and competence.
D. Review the interview, the validity of the plans, and the next step.
E. None of the above.

10.5   In emergency settings, the focus of the parent interview is

    A. Directly related to the parents' sense of control, frustration, and incompetence in the clinical situation.
    B. To assess the risk of danger and to establish a safe and protective environment for the child.
    C. To assess the child's medical care.
    D. To obtain factual and impressionistic information.
    E. All of the above.

C H A P T E R   1 1

Initial and Diagnostic Family Interviews

Select the single best response for each question.

11.1   The diagnostic family interview is commonly divided into three segments: 1) social stage, 2) multidimensional inquiry into the presenting problem, and 3) exploration of the structure and developmental phase of the family. During the *multidimensional inquiry stage* of the initial family interview

    A. The clinician initiates the engagement by serving as host to the family.
    B. The clinician does not yet address the presenting problem.
    C. The clinician should be prepared to encounter family resistance to broadening the focus of the discussion.
    D. The clinical assessment of the family's developmental level is of primary importance.
    E. The clinician focuses on the functional adequacy of various family subsystems.

11.2   Which of the following is *not* considered an accepted therapist function during family assessment?

    A. Understanding the roles of the different family members.
    B. Uncovering explicit and implicit family rules.
    C. Determining the family's typical problem-solving strategies.
    D. Understanding the nature of boundaries, splits, and alliances among family members.
    E. Allying with healthier family members during discussions with less healthy members.

11.3   The family life-cycle stage of "becoming three" is best defined as

    A. Establishment of a common household by two adults.
    B. Development of parental identity.
    C. Arrival and inclusion of the first child.
    D. Exit of the oldest child from the family during late adolescence.
    E. Death of a spouse.

11.4   Which of the following is *not* one of Minuchin's (1974) major areas of family assessment?

    A. The family structure.
    B. The family financial status.
    C. The family system's flexibility.
    D. The family life context.
    E. The family developmental stage.

11.5   Which of the following family rating scales, widely used in research, measures the social climate of all types of families, with subscales in the areas of family cohesion, expressiveness, conflict, independence, and achievement?

A. The Family Environment Scale.
B. The Card Sorting Procedure.
C. The Family Adaptability Cohesion Evaluation Scale.
D. The Beavers-Timberlawn Family Evaluation Scale.
E. The Family Assessment Device.

CHAPTER 12

Diagnostic Interviews

Select the single best response for each question.

12.1 According to Angold and Fisher (1999), clinician diagnoses are potentially fraught with numerous biases. All of the following are examples of such biases *except*

A. Making diagnoses before all relevant information is collected.
B. Collecting information selectively when confirming and/or ruling out a diagnosis.
C. Not systematically collecting and organizing information.
D. Not permitting one's special expertise to influence diagnostic assessment.
E. Assuming correlations in symptoms and illnesses that in reality are spurious or nonexistent.

12.2 *Construct validity* is defined as

A. How well a category as defined appears to describe a recognized illness.
B. Whether a category has meaning in terms of what it is designed to describe.
C. How well a category predicts a pertinent aspect of care.
D. How internally consistent a measure is.
E. How often different interviewers assign the same diagnosis.

12.3 Which of the statements concerning reliability is *false?*

A. Reliability includes how often different interviewers assign the same diagnosis.
B. Diagnostic tools need to be reliable in order to be useful.
C. Reliability ensures validity.
D. Reliability includes how internally consistent the measure is.
E. Reliability encompasses how consistently respondents report the same symptoms or diagnoses over time.

12.4 Which of the following statements concerning assessment of a diagnostic instrument's ability to detect cases is *true?*

A. *Sensitivity* is the percentage of individuals in a sample who have the disorder who are accurately identified by the interview.
B. *Predictive value positive* is the percentage of individuals in the defined sample positively identified by the interview who actually have the disorder.
C. *Specificity* is the percentage of individuals in a sample who do not have the disorder who are accurately identified by the interview as not having the disorder.
D. *Predictive value negative* is the percentage of individuals in the defined sample identified as not having the disorder by the interview who in fact do not have the disorder.
E. All of the above.

12.5 Although a number of structured diagnostic interviews are available for assessment of psychiatric illnesses in youth, these instruments have limitations. Examples of such limitations include all of the following *except*

A. Children may underreport new or unusual phenomena.
B. Children may lack the requisite attention span.
C. Children may lack the abstract awareness to understand the concepts.
D. Children may not be aware of the concept being described.
E. Children may lack the necessary verbal skills.

C H A P T E R   1 3

Rating Scales

Select the single best response for each question.

13.1 The *reliability* of a rating instrument

    A. Is equivalent to random error.
    B. Refers to the consistency with which an instrument measures a construct in the same way every time.
    C. Pertains to whether the instrument accurately assesses what it was designed to measure.
    D. Is inversely proportional to the validity of the instrument.
    E. Is reduced when the measured construct changes over time.

13.2 Which of the following is the best example of a broad-band rating scale?

    A. Conners Rating Scale—Revised.
    B. Children's Depression Inventory.
    C. Hopelessness Scale for Children.
    D. Child Behavior Checklist.
    E. ADHD Rating Scale–IV.

13.3 All of the following statements pertaining to broad-band rating scales are correct *except*

    A. They include measurements of both internalizing and externalizing behaviors.
    B. They assess a variety of clinical problems.
    C. They may be lengthy and cumbersome to complete.
    D. They assess for both breadth and depth of pathology in all clinical domains.
    E. They are best used to identify problems that will require further evaluation.

13.4 The Conners Rating Scale—Revised

    A. Includes parent, teacher, and youth self-report versions.
    B. Mostly assesses internalizing behaviors.
    C. Includes some abbreviated versions, but only for youth self-report.
    D. Has no mechanism for assessing common comorbid conditions.
    E. Is most useful for initial assessment in its abbreviated version.

13.5 Which of the following scales measuring internalizing symptoms is clinician-administered rather than self-reported?

    A. Beck Depression Inventory.
    B. Children's Depression Inventory.
    C. Children's Depression Rating Scale.
    D. Beck Hopelessness Scale.
    E. Hopelessness Scale for Children.

CHAPTER 14

Psychological and Neuropsychological Testing

Select the single best response for each question.

14.1   Which of the following statements concerning intelligence tests is *true*?

   A. Intelligence test scores vary widely for children over the age of 5 years.
   B. IQ scores are strong predictors of overall adjustment.
   C. IQ scores are strongly associated with academic achievement.
   D. All of the above.
   E. None of the above.

14.2   According to DSM-IV-TR (American Psychiatric Association 2000), an individual is identified as being mentally retarded if, in addition to being functionally impaired, he or she has a standardized IQ score below

   A. 90.
   B. 70.
   C. 50.
   D. 30.
   E. None of the above.

14.3   Which of the following instruments measures intellectual and cognitive functioning in children and adolescents?

   A. McCarthy Scales of Children's Abilities.
   B. Kaufman Assessment Battery for Children.
   C. Leiter International Performance Scale—Revised.
   D. Differential Abilities Scale.
   E. All of the above.

14.4   All of the following are measures of socioemotional functioning in children and adolescents *except*

   A. Gestalt Closure Test.
   B. Children's Apperception Test.
   C. Rorschach Inkblot Test.
   D. Sentence-completion test.
   E. Human Figure Drawing.

C H A P T E R   1 5

Laboratory and Diagnostic Testing

Select the single best response for each question.

15.1   In a study conducted by Sheline and Kehr (1990), the use of screening tests in psychiatric inpatients led to changes in clinical management in what percentage of cases?

   A. 1%.
   B. 6%.
   C. 10%.
   D. 14%.
   E. None of the above.

15.2   Laboratory tests recommended as part of a comprehensive examination or premedication workup include all of the following *except*

   A. Complete blood count (CBC).
   B. Urinalysis.
   C. Thyroid panel.
   D. Liver function tests.
   E. Blood urea nitrogen (BUN).

15.3   Which of the following thyroid disorders has been reported to be associated with attention-deficit/hyperactivity disorder (ADHD)–like symptoms?

   A. Hyperthyroidism.
   B. Syndrome of resistance to thyroid hormone.
   C. Hypothyroidism.
   D. All of the above.
   E. None of the above.

15.4   For patients who attempt suicide by drug overdose, recommended medical/laboratory tests depend on the specific substance taken. Which of the following recommendations is *incorrect*?

   A. Blood toxicology workup for overdose on illegal substances.
   B. Liver function test for acetaminophen overdose.
   C. Serum electrolytes for aspirin overdose.
   D. Electrocardiogram (ECG) for selective serotonin reuptake inhibitor (SSRI) overdose.
   E. None of the above.

15.5 Peer-reviewed articles support the use of single-photon emission computed tomography (SPECT) to rule out which of the following disorders in children?

A. ADHD.
B. Wilson's disease.
C. Seizure disorder.
D. Prader-Willi syndrome.
E. None of the above.

C H A P T E R   1 6
Clinical Genomic Testing

Select the single best response for each question.

16.1   Which of the following statements concerning the cytochrome P450 *2D6* gene is *false?*

    A. It is primarily responsible for the metabolism of many psychotropic medications such as fluoxetine, paroxetine, and selected tricyclic antidepressants.
    B. It is located on the long arm of chromosome 22.
    C. Unlike other cytochrome P450 genes, it has few polymorphisms.
    D. It metabolizes codeine.
    E. None of the above.

16.2   Polymorphisms associated with which of the following dopamine transporter or receptor genes have been found in selected families with a well-documented history of schizophrenia?

    A. Dopamine transporter gene.
    B. Dopamine receptor 2 gene.
    C. Dopamine receptor 3 gene.
    D. Dopamine receptor 4 gene.
    E. None of the above.

16.3   Polymorphisms of the serotonin transporter (*5HTT*) gene have been reported to be associated with all of the following *except*

    A. Obsessive-compulsive disorder.
    B. Suicidal behavior in depressed patients.
    C. Autism.
    D. Attention-deficit/hyperactivity disorder (ADHD).
    E. Increased fear- and anxiety-related symptoms.

16.4   Polymorphisms of the tryptophan hydroxylase (*TPH*) gene have been linked to all of the following *except*

    A. Suicidal behavior.
    B. Bipolar disorder.
    C. Early smoking initiation.
    D. Panic disorder.
    E. Alcohol abuse.

16.5   Critical elements of medical testing that also apply to genomic testing include all of the following *except*

    A. There should be adequate informed consent.
    B. Testing need not be voluntary.
    C. Test results must be accurate.
    D. Information obtained from the test must provide some potential medical or psychological benefit.
    E. The patient should be provided with information on both benefits and risks.

C H A P T E R   1 7

Diagnosis and Diagnostic Formulation

Select the single best response for each question.

17.1   The psychiatric formulation of a child's case

    A. Must simultaneously consider biological, social, developmental, and psychological contributing factors.

    B. Requires access to one or two sources of information.

    C. Is a relatively simple process.

    D. May not require consideration of social factors in some cases.

    E. Requires that the child be viewed as separate and distinct from his or her family network.

17.2   Which of the following statements regarding the Diagnostic and Statistical Manual (DSM) is *true?*

    A. The DSM clarifies the etiology for most disorders.

    B. The DSM incorporates multiple theoretical paradigms in defining disorder caseness.

    C. The use of DSM typically results in low comorbidity of psychiatric diagnoses in the child population.

    D. The DSM requires descriptive symptomatology to qualify for diagnosis using established criteria.

    E. Resultant DSM diagnoses link to precise and effective treatments.

17.3   Which of the following statements concerning DSM-IV-TR (2000) developmental disorders is *false?*

    A. The category includes pervasive developmental disorders and autism.

    B. The category does not include mental retardation.

    C. Diagnoses in this category are coded on Axis II.

    D. Typically, disorders in this category are characterized by an uneven or deviant developmental profile.

    E. These disorders commonly co-occur with other conditions.

17.4   In cataloging the relevant biological features of a child's case, important factors to consider include all of the following *except*

    A. Family genetic history.

    B. Early caregiving practices.

    C. Language disorder history in first-degree relatives.

    D. Early childhood meningitis.

    E. Malnutrition.

17.5   Which of the following statements concerning psychodynamic formulations is *false*?

A. The presence of unconscious functioning is assumed.
B. Unconscious internal conflicts typically contribute to symptom formation.
C. Symptoms have psychological meaning to the child.
D. Presenting problems are driven to expression within the transference relationship with the therapist.
E. Nondynamic factors are extraneous to the formulation.

CHAPTER 18

Presentation of Findings and Recommendations

Select the single best response for each question.

18.1   The main purposes of the postassessment or "informing" interview in regard to a child or adolescent patient include which of the following?

    A. Sharing the clinician's observation with the child's parents.

    B. Elaborating further on parental feelings and perceptions.

    C. Discussing the clinician's recommendations.

    D. Arriving at a plan that will be helpful to the child and the family.

    E. All of the above.

18.2   Which of the following statements concerning confidentiality in children and adolescents is *false?*

    A. Confidentiality is qualitatively different for younger children than for adolescents.

    B. The clinician can promise confidentiality to a child with the proviso that information that is potentially self-destructive or destructive to others will be shared with those who may protect the child.

    C. It is usually necessary to include younger children in the postdiagnostic interview.

    D. The issues of confidentiality are of greater importance to adolescent patients than they are for adult patients.

    E. None of the above.

18.3   Factors that are relevant to a family's remaining in therapy include all of the following *except*

    A. The therapist's activity and directiveness.

    B. The family's ability to influence the consultation.

    C. The congruence between the family's expectations and the therapist's response.

    D. The severity of the child's psychiatric disorder.

    E. The family's perception that they are active participants in the therapeutic process.

CHAPTER 19

Mental Retardation

Select the single best response for each question.

19.1   DSM-IV-TR (American Psychiatric Association 2000) criteria require an IQ score in which of the following ranges for a diagnosis of "severe mental retardation"?

   A. Below 20–25.
   B. Between 20–25 and 35–40.
   C. Between 35–40 and 50–55.
   D. Between 50–55 and 70.
   E. None of the above.

19.2   Data from the National Health Interview Survey for 1994–1995 (University of Minnesota 2000) indicate that the combined prevalence of mental retardation and developmental disabilities in the United States during that period was approximately what percentage of the population?

   A. 1.5%.
   B. 3%.
   C. 5%.
   D. 7%.
   E. 9%.

19.3   Prader-Willi syndrome in children is characterized by all of the following *except*

   A. Obesity.
   B. Hypogonadism in males.
   C. Spasticity.
   D. Dysmorphic features.
   E. Hyperphagia.

19.4   DNA probes and molecular biology analyses have identified the q11–q12 region of chromosome 15 as the abnormal region of the human genome responsible for which of the following syndromes?

   A. Prader-Willi syndrome and Angelman's syndrome.
   B. Angelman's syndrome and fragile X syndrome.
   C. Prader-Willi syndrome and fragile X syndrome.
   D. Prader-Willi syndrome and Williams syndrome.
   E. Fragile X syndrome and Rett's disorder.

19.5　The most common inherited form of mental retardation is

　　A.　Angelman's syndrome.
　　B.　Rett's disorder.
　　C.　Williams syndrome.
　　D.　Prader-Willi syndrome.
　　E.　Fragile X syndrome.

19.6　Current estimates of the prevalence of schizophrenia in individuals with mental retardation are in the range of

　　A.　1%–3%.
　　B.　3%–5%.
　　C.　5%–8%.
　　D.　8%–10%.
　　E.　10%–12%.

CHAPTER 20

Autistic Disorder

Select the single best response for each question.

20.1   Which of the following is an essential characteristic of infantile autism, as proposed by Rutter (1968)?

   A. Onset before age 30 months.
   B. Bizarre motor behavior.
   C. Impaired language.
   D. Lack of social interest and responsiveness.
   E. All of the above.

20.2   All of the following are pervasive developmental disorders *except*

   A. Autistic disorder.
   B. Mental retardation.
   C. Rett's disorder.
   D. Childhood disintegrative disorder.
   E. Asperger's disorder.

20.3   A common comorbid medical condition noted in patients with autism is epilepsy. Which of the following statements is *true*?

   A. The risk of epilepsy in patients with autism is highest during late adolescence.
   B. A prospective study of epilepsy in children with autistic spectrum disorders found a rate of 5%.
   C. The most common type of epilepsy is generalized or grand mal seizures.
   D. Males with autism have seizures more frequently than do females with autism.
   E. None of the above.

20.4   All of the following psychopharmacological agents have been reported to decrease autistic symptoms *except*

   A. Fluoxetine.
   B. Fluvoxamine.
   C. Quetiapine.
   D. Venlafaxine.
   E. Sertraline.

20.5   Which of the following factors has consistently been shown to be related to outcome in autistic patients?

   A. Age at onset.
   B. Family history of mental illness.
   C. IQ.
   D. Perinatal complications.
   E. Birth weight.

C H A P T E R   2 1

Other Pervasive Developmental Disorders

Select the single best response for each question.

21.1 Which of the following symptoms is *least* likely to be present in Asperger's disorder?

A. Impairment in nonverbal social interactions.
B. Impairment in peer relationships.
C. General delay in language development.
D. Lack of social or emotional reciprocity.
E. Restricted repetitive or stereotyped patterns of behavior or interests.

21.2 In regard to differences between Asperger's disorder and autistic disorder, all of the following clinical and research findings are correct *except*

A. Asperger's disorder may be associated with a higher verbal IQ than found in high-functioning autism (Klin et al. 1995; Ramberg et al. 1996).
B. On the Wechsler Intelligence Scale for Children—Revised, individuals with Asperger's disorder had good verbal ability and troughs on Object Assembly and Coding, whereas those with autistic disorder had a peak on Block Design (Ehlers et al. 1997).
C. On the Rorschach inkblot test, adolescents with Asperger's had lower levels of disorganized thinking than did those with high-functioning autism (Ghaziuddin et al. 1995).
D. In a study examining the development of theory of mind in children with autism and Asperger's disorder, Asperger patients performed better than autism patients on false belief, belief term comprehension, and belief term expression tasks (Ziatas et al. 1998).
E. Asperger patients are more likely than autism patients to be argumentative, aggressive, and condescending.

21.3 In Hagberg and Witt-Engerström's (1986) four-stage model of the course of neurological deterioration in Rett's disorder, the *rapid developmental regression stage*

A. Often occurs during school age or early adolescence.
B. Occurs between the ages of 6 months and 1.5 years, with a median age of 10–11 months.
C. Usually occurs at age 1–2 years and lasts for 13–19 months.
D. Usually occurs at age 3–4 years but can be delayed and can persist for many years or even decades.
E. Marks the period of slowest deterioration of all stages.

21.4   Which of the following statements concerning childhood disintegrative disorder is *true*?

    A. Childhood disintegrative disorder is a common condition.
    B. It usually develops during the first year of life.
    C. The developmental regression, once initiated, typically progresses over a period of several years.
    D. Children rarely regain any language ability once developmental regression has occurred.
    E. It is associated with a high prevalence of epilepsy.

21.5   The DSM-IV-TR (American Psychiatric Association 2000) subtype *residual autism* of pervasive developmental disorder not otherwise specified (PDDNOS) is exemplified by which of the following?

    A. Individuals who "almost but not quite" meet the full criteria for autism.
    B. Individuals who have a history of autism but who currently do not meet full criteria.
    C. Individuals who "almost but not quite" meet criteria for Asperger's disorder.
    D. Individuals who show mixed features of autism and Asperger's disorder.
    E. Individuals with comorbid medical or neurological disorders associated with autism.

C H A P T E R   2 2

Developmental Disorders of Learning, Motor Skills, and Communication

Select the single best response for each question.

22.1 Which of the following statements concerning the clinical presentation of learning disorders is *false*?

   A. Reading disorder occurs in 2%–20% of children.
   B. Reading disorder accounts for up to 80% of all children diagnosed with a learning disorder.
   C. An equal proportion of boys and girls are diagnosed with a reading disorder.
   D. Disorder of written expression is more common in boys than in girls.
   E. Mathematics disorder is reported to occur in 1%–6% of school-age children.

22.2 All of the following statements concerning developmental coordination disorder are correct *except*

   A. The disorder occurs in up to 6% of 5- to 11-year-olds.
   B. The clumsiness associated with this disorder can lead to peer teasing.
   C. Children with developmental coordination disorder seldom have associated delays of other developmental milestones.
   D. Comorbid conditions such as attention-deficit/hyperactivity disorder (ADHD) are frequently seen in children with developmental coordination disorder.
   E. The coordination deficits may continue throughout life.

22.3 In language, *morphology* is defined as

   A. A language's sound system and accompanying rules governing the combination of sounds.
   B. The system that governs the structure and formation of words in a language.
   C. The system that governs the order and combination of words to form sentences.
   D. The system that governs the meaning of words and sentences.
   E. The system that combines the language components into functional and socially appropriate communication.

22.4 Which of the following communication disorders disproportionately affects males?

   A. Developmental (versus acquired) expressive language disorder.
   B. Mixed receptive–expressive language disorder.
   C. Phonological disorder.
   D. Stuttering.
   E. All of the above.

22.5 Which of the following statements concerning the etiology of communication disorders is *false*?

A. The etiology is primarily due to family environment and sociological factors.
B. Exposure to intrauterine teratogens may adversely affect language development.
C. Anoxia and asphyxia have been implicated in the development of communication disorders.
D. Important environmental risk factors for the development of communication disorders include poverty and abuse or neglect.
E. Early childhood risk factors that have been implicated in communication disorders include persistent otitis media and other childhood illnesses.

CHAPTER 23

Schizophrenia and Other Psychotic Disorders

Select the single best response for each question.

23.1 The diagnosis of schizophrenia with childhood onset

    A. Is a common presentation for this disorder.
    B. Is five times more likely in females than in males.
    C. Requires no mood disorder exclusion.
    D. Can be made when signs of disturbance have been present for at least 3 months.
    E. May have a prevalence of less than 1 in 1,000.

23.2 In regard to National Institute of Mental Health studies comparing patients with childhood-onset schizophrenia and patients with adult-onset schizophrenia, all of the following findings are correct *except*

    A. Childhood-onset patients showed greater delay in language development than did adult-onset patients.
    B. Childhood-onset patients evidenced more disruptive behavior disorders than did adult-onset patients.
    C. Childhood-onset patients evidenced more learning disorders than did adult-onset patients.
    D. Childhood-onset patients evidenced few motor stereotypies.
    E. Childhood-onset schizophrenia appears to represent a more malignant form of the disorder.

23.3 Which phase of illness in schizophrenic patients is best described by the following definition: "A 1- to 6-month (or longer) period when symptoms of hallucinations, delusions, thought disorder, or disorganized behavior are predominant?"

    A. Prodrome.
    B. Acute phase.
    C. Recovery phase.
    D. Residual phase.
    E. Chronicity.

23.4 Which of the following statements concerning the differential diagnosis of childhood psychotic disorders is *true*?

A. The diagnostic criteria for schizophreniform disorder require an illness duration of less than 6 months.
B. Once a diagnosis of schizophreniform disorder is made, a diagnosis of schizophrenia can never be given.
C. A diagnosis of schizophreniform disorder requires the presence of a decline in function.
D. Brief psychotic disorder requires a symptom duration of at least 1 month but no more than 6 months.
E. The diagnosis of psychotic disorder not otherwise specified is very rare in the hospitalized adolescent population.

23.5 Magnetic resonance imaging (MRI) studies in children with schizophrenia have reported all of the following findings *except*

A. Decreases in total cerebral volume.
B. Cerebral asymmetry.
C. Decreases in ventricular volume.
D. Increases in temporal lobe volume.
E. Decreases in midsagittal thalamic area.

CHAPTER 24

Mood Disorders in Prepubertal Children

Select the single best response for each question.

24.1 Childhood mood disorders are often underdiagnosed or misdiagnosed for which of the following reasons?

   A. The belief, on the part of some clinicians, that a child's immature superego and personality structure do not permit the development of a mood disorder.
   B. Many children lack the capacity to express their emotions verbally.
   C. Many children present with somatic complaints that are diagnosed as physical illness.
   D. Parents who are bipolar are often underdiagnosed.
   E. All of the above.

24.2 Prepubertal children with major depression routinely present with atypical features. Symptoms consistent with such a presentation include all of the following *except*

   A. Hypersomnia.
   B. Weight loss.
   C. Psychomotor retardation.
   D. Mood reactivity.
   E. Increased appetite.

24.3 In contrast to manic adults, manic children usually present with all of the following symptoms *except*

   A. Irritability.
   B. Impulsivity.
   C. Euphoria.
   D. Depression.
   E. Inability to concentrate.

24.4 What proportion of children with major depressive episodes show signs of bipolar disorder by adolescence?

   A. One-quarter.
   B. One-third.
   C. One-half.
   D. Two-thirds.
   E. Three-fourths.

24.5   Which of the following statements concerning school-age children with mood disorders is *true?*

   A. They do not attempt suicide.
   B. They are unable to describe their symptoms.
   C. They tend not to somatize their symptoms.
   D. Mania is usually characterized by pressured speech.
   E. School performance is usually unaffected.

CHAPTER 25

Mood Disorders in Adolescents

Select the single best response for each question.

25.1 Commonly presenting symptoms of depression in adolescents include

A. Poor school performance.
B. Social withdrawal.
C. Substance abuse.
D. Conduct disorder.
E. All of the above.

25.2 Diagnosing bipolar disorder in adolescence may be challenging for all of the following reasons *except*

A. Presenting symptoms are often minor or major depression.
B. Severity of symptoms frequently results in hospitalization.
C. Because symptoms may build up gradually, they frequently are overlooked.
D. Inappropriate sexual behavior and other "atypical" presentation are common.
E. Serious conduct behaviors, such as vandalism, may mask underlying manic symptoms.

25.3 In a study by Carlson et al. (2000) comparing patients with early-onset (between the ages of 15 and 20 years) and adult-onset bipolar disorder, which of the following findings was reported?

A. Women predominated in the early-onset group.
B. More remissions occurred during follow-up in the early-onset group than in the adult-onset group.
C. Individuals in the early-onset group were more likely than those in the adult-onset group to have a substance use disorder.
D. Patients with early-onset bipolar disorder had an increased risk of mood-incongruent psychotic symptoms.
E. Depressive episodes occurred more frequently in the early-onset group.

25.4 Approximately 40%–70% of children and adolescents with major depressive disorder have a comorbid psychiatric disorder. All of the following are common comorbid conditions *except*

A. Eating disorders.
B. Anxiety disorders.
C. Dysthymic disorder.
D. Disruptive behavior disorder.
E. Substance use.

25.5 Common side effects of lithium treatment in children and adolescents include all of the following *except*

A. Diarrhea.
B. Tremor.
C. Leukopenia.
D. Fatigue.
E. Ataxia.

CHAPTER 26

Attention-Deficit/ Hyperactivity Disorder

Select the single best response for each question.

26.1 Which of the following is *not* one of the core symptom clusters of attention-deficit/hyperactivity disorder (ADHD) as identified in DSM-IV-TR (American Psychiatric Association 2000)?

A. Hyperactivity.
B. Inattention.
C. Impulsivity.
D. Disruptive behavior.
E. Distractibility.

26.2 Which of the following is *not* one of the DSM-IV-TR diagnostic criteria for ADHD?

A. Symptoms must have persisted for at least 6 months.
B. Symptoms must be evident in at least two different environments.
C. Symptoms must have been present before age 5 years.
D. Symptoms must be maladaptive in terms of functioning.
E. Symptoms cannot be accounted for by another DSM-IV-TR diagnosis (e.g., a pervasive developmental disorder).

26.3 Which of the following comorbid psychiatric disorders has been reported to occur most frequently in children diagnosed with ADHD?

A. Schizophrenia.
B. Oppositional defiant disorder.
C. Autism.
D. Bipolar disorder.
E. Panic disorder.

26.4 Which of the following statements concerning the epidemiology of ADHD is *false*?

A. The disorder seems to be more common in boys than in girls.
B. The prevalence reported in DSM-IV-TR is 3%–7% of school-age children.
C. ADHD is more common in school-age populations than in older populations.
D. Prevalence rates show little variation across cultures, countries, and settings (urban, suburban, and rural).
E. None of the above.

26.5 Which of the following statements concerning research findings on the course and duration of ADHD is *correct*?

A. At least some impairment from the disorder is present in most adolescents who were referred for clinical treatment as school-age children.
B. The disorder is generally episodic rather than chronic.
C. Inattention tends to remit over time, in contrast to hyperactivity, which is remarkably persistent.
D. Inattention symptoms may place a child at greater risk for the development of antisocial behavior.
E. None of the above.

26.6 The research literature supports the use of all of the following medications for ADHD *except*

A. Tricyclic antidepressants.
B. Psychostimulants.
C. Clonidine.
D. Bupropion.
E. Benzodiazepines.

C H A P T E R 2 7

Conduct Disorder and Oppositional Defiant Disorder

Select the single best response for each question.

27.1   Which of the following statements regarding the diagnoses of conduct disorder and oppositional defiant disorder (ODD) is *true?*

A. Children with these disorders are a distinct group that presents in a uniform and narrow fashion.
B. The relationship between conduct disorder and ODD is clearly defined.
C. The diagnosis of conduct disorder is controversial in child psychiatry.
D. ODD behaviors typically are preceded by more serious violations of age-appropriate behavioral norms.
E. Conduct disorder has been determined to be a biological condition.

27.2   All of the following statements regarding the prevalence of conduct disorder are correct *except*

A. The prevalence of conduct disorder is difficult to estimate because of variations in definition.
B. The prevalence is estimated as approximately 9% for males and 2% for females younger than 18 years.
C. The childhood-onset type of the disorder (onset before 10 years of age) is clearly much more common in males.
D. Individuals with adolescent-onset conduct disorder are much more likely to develop adult antisocial personality disorder than are those with childhood-onset conduct disorder.
E. Adolescent-onset conduct disorder is less likely than childhood-onset conduct disorder to involve a preponderance of males.

27.3   Which of the following statements regarding subtypes of conduct disorder is *true?*

A. Subtyping aggressive behavior into predatory and affective categories is not a useful distinction.
B. Predatory aggression is characterized by the presence of high levels of autonomic and emotional arousal with little apparent instrumental gain.
C. Children who demonstrate reactive aggression tend to be more delinquent than those demonstrating proactive aggression.
D. The process of subclassifying conduct disorder according to age at onset, degree of aggressivity, and extent of socialization has been completely validated.
E. The value of subtyping conduct disorder into childhood-onset and adolescent-onset variants is related to the prognostic significance of age at onset.

27.4 A biological factor associated with conduct disorder is

   A. Reduced novelty-seeking trait.
   B. A history of maternal smoking during pregnancy.
   C. Anxious temperament.
   D. Reduced rates of expression of the *L/L* variant of the serotonin transporter gene.
   E. Elevated harm-avoidance trait.

27.5 All of the following statements concerning treatment of youngsters with conduct disorder are correct *except*

   A. Treatment may take place in a variety of different long-term and short-term programs in outpatient, inpatient, and residential settings.
   B. Cognitive-behavioral approaches include improvement in problem-solving skills, impulse control, and anger management.
   C. Family therapy is not an effective treatment modality in conduct disorder patients.
   D. Parent management training focuses on modifying coercive parent–child interactions that encourage child antisocial behaviors.
   E. When used, pharmacotherapy commonly targets aggression in the conduct disorder population.

C H A P T E R   2 8

Conduct and Antisocial Disorders in Adolescence

Select the single best response for each question.

28.1 Which of the following statements concerning the diagnosis of conduct disorder is *false?*

　A. The DSM-IV (American Psychiatric Association 1994) definition of conduct disorder is similar to that found in DSM-III-R (American Psychiatric Association 1987).

　B. The child must have manifested five or more of a list of undesirable behaviors in the previous 6 months.

　C. A list of 15 undesirable behaviors is grouped into four categories.

　D. All of the undesirable behaviors defining conduct disorders occur as part of many other diagnoses.

　E. A study of youth from U.S. communities (Lahey et al. 1999) documented a strong association between very early behavior problems and subsequent serious aggressive behaviors.

28.2 Which of the following statements concerning the clinical presentation of conduct and antisocial disorders in adolescent is *true?*

　A. Mania in adolescence can mimic attention-deficit/hyperactivity disorder (ADHD), oppositional defiant disorder, and conduct disorder.

　B. Studies of adult psychiatric patients as well as studies of psychopathology in violent delinquent adolescents demonstrate little relationship between violence and serious psychopathology.

　C. Fewer than 20% of arrested male juveniles have drugs or alcohol in their bloodstreams.

　D. ADHD was rarely found to coexist in most cases of early-onset conduct disorder.

　E. Less than 25% of children with ADHD also manifest evidence of oppositional defiant disorder or conduct disorder.

28.3 In animal studies, which chemical has been reported to be of importance in the development of normal bonding?

　A. Glutamate.

　B. Oxytocin.

　C. Progesterone.

　D. Gamma-aminobutyric acid (GABA).

　E. Estrogen.

28.4   According to Kazdin (2001), treatment modalities found to produce positive behavioral change in children with conduct disorder include all of the following *except*

A. Parent management training.
B. Group therapy.
C. Cognitive problem-solving skills training.
D. Multisystemic therapy.
E. Functional family therapy.

28.5   Which of the following statements concerning children who have been diagnosed with conduct disorder is *true*?

A. A majority go on to commit aggressive antisocial acts in adulthood.
B. The overall adult adjustment is often good.
C. Suicide and other forms of violent death are common.
D. Many go on to stable marriages after they outgrow symptoms.
E. Most have satisfactory job histories.

CHAPTER 29

Separation Anxiety Disorder and Generalized Anxiety Disorder

Select the single best response for each question.

29.1 Separation anxiety

    A. Begins at age 18 months and peaks at age 30 months.
    B. Is a normative part of development.
    C. Usually indicates the presence of a disorder.
    D. Symptoms are seldom subclinically present in the pediatric population.
    E. Is rarely persistent and excessive.

29.2 Which of the following DSM-IV-TR (American Psychiatric Association 2000) criteria is *not* required in order to make a diagnosis of generalized anxiety disorder (GAD) in children?

    A. Excessive anxiety and worry for at least a 6-month period.
    B. Difficulty controlling the worry.
    C. Three or more associated physiological symptoms (restlessness, fatigue, difficulty concentrating, irritability, muscle tension, or sleep disturbance).
    D. The focus of the worry is not related to another Axis I condition.
    E. Presence of clinically significant distress or impairment.

29.3 Which of the following statements regarding the epidemiology of GAD and SAD is *true*?

    A. SAD is more prevalent among older children.
    B. GAD is more prevalent among younger children.
    C. Rates of SAD increase with age.
    D. Rates of SAD and GAD do not vary with age.
    E. Rates of GAD increase with age.

29.4 Which of the following statements about temperament and its contributing role to childhood anxiety is *false?*

A. Approximately 20% of healthy infants are born with traits that predispose them to become highly reactive in novel environments (Kagan and Snidman 1999).
B. Kagan (1994) described the temperamental characteristic of behavioral inhibition as a child's tendency to approach unfamiliar or novel situations with distress, restraint, or avoidance.
C. Behavioral inhibition appears to be a highly unstable temperamental trait.
D. Children with behavioral inhibition may be differentiated from non–behaviorally inhibited children through neurophysiological markers (Kagan et al. 1988).
E. Children who are identified as shy may be more prone to anxiety symptoms than those who are not (Biederman et al. 1995).

29.5 The use of selective serotonin reuptake inhibitors (SSRIs) in the treatment of childhood anxiety disorders

A. Is considered a second-line choice (after benzodiazepines).
B. Has been supported by the results of several recent randomized, placebo-controlled trials.
C. Should usually continue indefinitely once initiated.
D. Has resulted in no documented side effects.
E. Has resulted in minimal clinical benefit over placebo.

CHAPTER 30

Obsessive-Compulsive Disorder

Select the single best response for each question.

30.1   According to studies conducted by Geller et al. (1998) and Swedo et al. (1989), which of the following epidemiological findings related to obsessive-compulsive disorder (OCD) is *false*?

   A. Girls tended to have an earlier age at onset.
   B. In young children, there was a male predominance (male-to-female ratio: 3 to 2).
   C. The mean age at onset was 10 years.
   D. Children with early-onset OCD were more likely to have a family member with OCD.
   E. In adolescence, the gender distribution between girls and boys with OCD was about equal.

30.2   Which of the following is *not* a proposed subtype of OCD in children?

   A. Early-onset OCD.
   B. Late-onset OCD.
   C. Tic-related OCD.
   D. Streptococcal-precipitated OCD.
   E. None of the above.

30.3   Several lines of neuroscience research have implicated, as a cause for OCD, a dysfunction in which brain structure?

   A. Hippocampus.
   B. Amygdala.
   C. Basal ganglia.
   D. Dorsal lateral prefrontal cortex.
   E. Substantia nigra.

30.4   Recent research supports the addition of which of the following pharmacological agents as an appropriate augmentation to a selective serotonin reuptake inhibitor (SSRI)?

   A. Lithium.
   B. Imipramine.
   C. Lamotrigine.
   D. Bupropion.
   E. Risperidone.

30.5 In the largest and most recent systematic follow-up study of children with OCD being treated with SSRIs and behavior therapy (Leonard et al. 1993), what percentage still met diagnostic criteria for OCD 2–7 years after initial presentation?

A. 17%.
B. 28%.
C. 43%.
D. 68%.
E. 82%.

C H A P T E R   3 1

Specific Phobia, Panic Disorder, Social Phobia, and Selective Mutism

Select the single best response for each question.

31.1   To which of the following disorders does the DSM-IV-TR (American Psychiatric Association 2000) definition "a marked and persistent fear that is excessive or unreasonable, cued by the presence or anticipation of a specific object or situation" apply?

    A. Social phobia.
    B. Selective mutism.
    C. Specific phobia.
    D. Panic disorder.
    E. Anxiety disorder not otherwise specified.

31.2   All of the following statements regarding panic disorder are correct *except*

    A. Panic attacks are the hallmark of panic disorder.
    B. Panic disorder may occur with or without agoraphobia.
    C. Children with early development of separation anxiety disorder are at increased risk of later developing panic disorder.
    D. Symptoms, course of illness, and associated complicating conditions in children with panic disorder are very different from those in adults with panic disorder.
    E. Panic disorder may develop at any age during childhood or later.

31.3   Individuals with social phobia commonly fear which of the following social situations?

    A. Public speaking or performing.
    B. Attending social gatherings.
    C. Dealing with authorities.
    D. Asking for directions.
    E. All of the above.

31.4 In regard to the prevalence of selective mutism in children, which of the following statements is *true*?

A. Prevalence estimates in children range from 3% to 5%.
B. Selective mutism symptoms that occur upon starting school are likely to be unremitting.
C. Variability in prevalence estimates may be due to vagueness in the DSM regarding the level of impairment required to meet diagnostic criteria.
D. Scandinavian prevalence studies have reported lower rates of selective mutism than have U.S. studies among school-age children.
E. Variability in prevalence estimates is unlikely to be related to differences in the consistent application of diagnostic criteria in study populations.

31.5 Which of the following descriptions refers to a *top-down* family genetic study of anxiety disorders?

A. The evaluation of the prevalence of anxiety disorders in the offspring of adult probands.
B. The evaluation of the prevalence of anxiety disorders in adult relatives of child probands.
C. The longitudinal evaluation of young offspring of adult probands with anxiety disorders.
D. The comparison of rates of co-occurrence of anxiety disorders in monozygotic twins.
E. The comparison of rates of co-occurrence of anxiety disorders in dizygotic twins.

C H A P T E R   3 2

Pediatric Posttraumatic Stress Disorder

Select the single best response for each question.

32.1   In assessing a child for posttraumatic stress disorder (PTSD), clinicians should do all of the following *except*

A. Establish that the incident actually occurred.
B. Take children's self-reports of trauma at face value.
C. Supplement children's self-reports with histories from parents and others.
D. Remember that children's recollections may be influenced by others.
E. Use a neutral questioning stance.

32.2   Stimuli directly or indirectly related to a traumatic event that provoke conditioned responses are known as

A. Traumatic dreams.
B. Reenactment behavior.
C. Traumatic play.
D. Traumatic reminders.
E. None of the above.

32.3   Traumatized children frequently have symptoms of disorders other than PTSD. In addition to true comorbidity, spurious comorbidity with PTSD can result from 1) overlap between criteria sets and 2) confounding similar symptoms of other diagnoses with those of PTSD. Which of the following disorders overlaps with or has symptoms similar to those of PTSD?

A. Attention-deficit/hyperactivity disorder (ADHD).
B. Oppositional defiant disorder.
C. Major depressive disorder.
D. Generalized anxiety disorder.
E. All of the above.

32.4   Important principles in the psychotherapeutic treatment of children with PTSD include all of the following *except*

A. Reexposing the individual to traumatic cues under safe conditions.
B. Allowing the sessions to be unfocused so that unconscious material may be uncovered.
C. Keeping focused on the child's current dysfunction.
D. Being diligent about continually rethinking the symptom picture.
E. Directing the therapy to facilitate higher levels of adaptation and coping.

32.5   Which of the following antidepressants has been approved by the U.S. Food and Drug Administration
        (FDA) for the treatment of PTSD in adults and is often used to treat PTSD in children and
        adolescents?

        A. Bupropion.
        B. Nefazodone.
        C. Imipramine.
        D. Duloxetine.
        E. Paroxetine.

CHAPTER 33

Feeding and Eating Disorders of Infancy and Early Childhood

Select the single best response for each question.

33.1   All of the following statements concerning feeding disorders in infants are correct *except*

   A. Up to 25% of otherwise healthy infants and young children have feeding problems.
   B. Common feeding difficulties include eating too little or too much food, food refusal, restricted food preferences, and bizarre food habits.
   C. Severe feeding problems, such as refusal to eat or vomiting, have been reported to occur in 5%–10% of infants younger than 1 year of age.
   D. Very few studies have followed the natural history of feeding problems.
   E. Up to 80% of infants and young children with developmental handicaps have feeding problems.

33.2   *Failure to thrive*

   A. Is an uncommon problem in pediatrics.
   B. Is a term used to describe infants and young children who develop poor attachments to caregivers during infancy.
   C. Was initially researched as a dichotomous condition, differentiated as organic and nonorganic failure to thrive.
   D. Is diagnosed when a child's decelerated or arrested growth results in height and weight below the 25th percentile.
   E. Has a presentation strikingly different from that of the *hospitalism* syndrome of Rene Spitz.

33.3   The DSM-IV-TR (American Psychiatric Association 2000) diagnostic criteria for infantile anorexia include which of the following?

   A. The child's refusal to eat adequate amounts of food is of at least 1 month's duration.
   B. The onset of the food refusal occurs before 6 years of age.
   C. The infant communicates hunger signals and evidences interest in food but shows little interest in exploration and/or interaction with the caregiver.
   D. The infant shows little growth deficiency.
   E. The food refusal may follow a traumatic event.

33.4   All of the following statements regarding posttraumatic feeding disorder are correct *except*

   A. Posttraumatic feeding disorder can occur at any age of development, from infancy to adulthood.
   B. The disorder is characterized by the sudden onset of total or partial food refusal.
   C. The condition has been reported in children who have undergone intubation or the insertion of nasogastric feeding tubes.
   D. Some children may refuse liquids but eat solids.
   E. Despite food refusal, feeding tends to be an apathetic process, with the child demonstrating neither emotional excitement nor emotional distress.

33.5   Which of the following statements regarding the condition *pica* is *true?*

   A. The diagnosis requires that a child demonstrate persistent eating of nonnutritive substances for a period of at least 6 months.
   B. The diagnosis would be appropriate in a 6-month-old child who often mouths nonnutritive objects.
   C. The diagnosis should be made when the ingestion is considered appropriate to the developmental level.
   D. Young children with pica often eat paint, plaster, paper, strings, hair, and cloth.
   E. Lead poison is no longer considered a common complication to pica.

C H A P T E R   3 4

Infant and Childhood Obesity

Select the single best response for each question.

34.1   The prevalence of obesity in early childhood is not nearly as well studied as the prevalence of obesity in adulthood. However, the few studies that have been conducted indicate the prevalence of obesity in preschool children to be in the range of

    A. 0–5%.
    B. 5%–10%.
    C. 10%–15%.
    D. 15%–20%.
    E. 20%–25%.

34.2   According to a report by the Centers for Disease Control and Prevention (2002), the prevalence of obesity in children between the ages of 6 and 19 years is in the range of

    A. 2%–5%.
    B. 6%–8%.
    C. 13%–14%.
    D. 21%–23%.
    E. 30%–33%.

34.3   According to the American Academy of Child and Adolescent Psychiatry (1997), if one parent is obese, children have what percentage chance of being obese?

    A. 10%.
    B. 30%.
    C. 40%.
    D. 50%.
    E. 70%.

34.4   Which of the following statements concerning the genetic/familial form of obesity is *true?*

    A. There is evidence of psychopathology in the child or parent.
    B. Evidence of nutritional misinformation is seen.
    C. The family history for obesity is negative.
    D. The obesity has a sudden onset, usually around ages 12–13 years.
    E. The child may have characteristics associated with "difficult temperament."

34.5 Which of the following statements regarding psychogenic obesity is *true*?

A. There is evidence of psychopathology in the child or parent.
B. There is no evidence of nutritional misinformation.
C. The family history for obesity is negative.
D. In one type, associated with traumatic separation from the primary caregiver, there is a sudden onset, usually before age 3 years.
E. All of the above.

CHAPTER 35

Anorexia Nervosa

Select the single best response for each question.

35.1 The DSM-IV-TR (American Psychiatric Association 2000) diagnostic criteria for anorexia nervosa include which of the following?

A. Body weight less than 50% of that expected.
B. Body height less than 85% of that expected.
C. Apathy to weight change.
D. Amenorrhea in postmenarcheal females.
E. Loss of interest in body habitus.

35.2 DSM-IV-TR distinguishes between two subtypes of anorexia nervosa. Which of the following statements regarding these subtypes is *false*?

A. The two subtypes are restricting and binge-eating/purging anorexia.
B. Those with restricting anorexia are more likely to have drug use disorders.
C. Those with binge-eating/purging anorexia are more likely to display impulse-control problems and mood lability.
D. Those with binge-eating/purging anorexia score higher on the Psychopathic Deviate, Depression, and Psychasthenia scales of the Minnesota Multiphasic Personality Inventory.
E. The majority of patients with restricting anorexia develop bulimic symptoms during the course of the disorder.

35.3 Common signs and symptoms associated with anorexia nervosa include which of the following?

A. Heat intolerance.
B. Tachycardia.
C. Diarrhea.
D. Breast engorgement.
E. Growth of lanugo hair.

35.4 Which of the following medical complications is *not* routinely associated with anorexia nervosa?

A. Arrhythmias.
B. Leukopenia.
C. Neurological abnormalities.
D. Decreased gastric motility.
E. Decreased bone mineral density.

35.5 Which of the following statements regarding the use of pharmacotherapy in the treatment of anorexia nervosa is *true*?

A. Medication has no adjunctive role.
B. Many psychotropic medications have been shown to effectively reverse the disorder.
C. Clomipramine and lithium have shown positive effects in clinical studies.
D. Fluoxetine may have a role in maintaining weight in weight-recovered anorexia patients.
E. Pharmacotherapy has been shown to be superior to combined medication–psychotherapy treatment in several studies.

CHAPTER 36

Bulimia Nervosa

Select the single best response for each question.

36.1 A number of studies have reported the prevalence of bulimia nervosa in young women to be in the range of

    A. 1%–4%.
    B. 5%–10%.
    C. 11%–15%.
    D. 16%–20%.
    E. 21%–25%.

36.2 DSM-IV-TR (American Psychiatric Association 2000) diagnostic criteria for bulimia nervosa include all of the following *except*

    A. The individual engages in recurrent episodes of binge eating.
    B. The individual engages in recurrent inappropriate compensatory behavior to prevent weight gain.
    C. Binge eating and inappropriate compensatory behaviors both occur, on average, at least weekly for 6 months.
    D. Self-evaluation is unduly influenced by body shape and weight.
    E. The disturbance does not occur exclusively during episodes of anorexia nervosa.

36.3 Compared with normal-weight individuals, persons with bulimia nervosa demonstrate elevations of which of the following neuropeptides and hormones?

    A. Neuropeptide Y.
    B. Cholecystokinin.
    C. Leptin.
    D. Cortisol.
    E. None of the above.

36.4 In a 5-year follow-up study by Barnett (1997), risk factors demonstrated to influence the etiology of bulimia nervosa included all of the following *except*

    A. Overinternalization of the value of thinness in women.
    B. Inordinate dissatisfaction with body form.
    C. Anxiety.
    D. Depression.
    E. Irrational beliefs and cognitions about thinness.

36.5   Which of the following antidepressants has been studied most extensively in bulimia nervosa and has been shown to be effective in its treatment?

A. Venlafaxine.
B. Mirtazapine.
C. Fluvoxamine.
D. Bupropion.
E. Fluoxetine.

C H A P T E R   3 7

Tic Disorders

Select the single best response for each question.

37.1   Which of the following statements regarding transient tic disorder is *true?*

    A.   Transient tics are very rare among prepubertal children.
    B.   Girls are more often affected than boys.
    C.   Transient tics run a waxing and waning course.
    D.   Transient tics most commonly involve the trunk and lower extremities.
    E.   Transient vocal tics are common.

37.2   All of the following statements regarding Tourette's syndrome are correct *except*

    A.   Chronic motor and phonic tic disorder was first described in 1885 by Georges Gilles de la Tourette.
    B.   Initial symptoms of Tourette's syndrome most frequently appear between the ages of 5 and 8 years.
    C.   Tic symptoms may wax and wane over time.
    D.   Vocal tics usually precede motor tics.
    E.   Children may be able to suppress tics for periods of time.

37.3   The most likely neuroanatomical substrate of Tourette's syndrome is

    A.   The thalamus.
    B.   The pituitary.
    C.   The prefrontal cortex.
    D.   The basal ganglia.
    E.   The amygdala.

37.4   Which of the following psychotropic agents is *least* likely to exacerbate tics?

    A.   Haloperidol.
    B.   L-dopa.
    C.   Dextroamphetamine.
    D.   Methylphenidate.
    E.   Cocaine.

37.5   Side effects of clonidine in the treatment of tic disorders include all of the following *except*

    A.   Sedation.
    B.   Irritability.
    C.   Dry mouth.
    D.   Cardiac arrhythmias.
    E.   Hypertension.

CHAPTER 38

Sleep Disorders in Infancy Through Adolescence

Select the single best response for each question.

38.1 Characteristics of non–rapid eye movement (NREM) sleep include all of the following *except*

A. Sleep spindles.
B. K complexes.
C. Active inhibition of muscle tone.
D. Delta waves.
E. Slowed and regular respiratory and heart rates.

38.2 In adults, sleep typically begins with which type of sleep, which occurs mostly during the first third of sleep?

A. REM.
B. NREM stage 1.
C. NREM stage 2.
D. NREM stage 3.
E. NREM stage 4.

38.3 All of the following are classified as dyssomnias in DSM-IV-TR (American Psychiatric Association 2000) *except*

A. Narcolepsy.
B. Sleep terror disorder.
C. Primary insomnia.
D. Primary hypersomnia.
E. Circadian rhythm sleep disorders.

38.4 Nighttime awakenings in infants have been categorized as either "signaled" or "self-soothing." Which of the following is a characteristic of self-soothing infants?

A. Self-soothers are more likely to be placed in their cribs while awake.
B. Self-soothers are more likely to use a sleep aid, such as a pacifier, to fall asleep.
C. Self-soothers may awaken for 3–5 minutes during the night but are able to fall asleep again on their own.
D. All of the above.
E. None of the above.

38.5   Common features of NREM parasomnias include all of the following *except*

A. A predominance in males.
B. A strong positive family history.
C. Retrograde amnesia for the event on the following morning.
D. Distress upon awakening.
E. None of the above.

38.6   Characteristics of narcolepsy include all of the following *except*

A. Irresistible attacks of NREM sleep.
B. Cataplexy.
C. Hypnagogic hallucinations.
D. Sleep paralysis.
E. None of the above.

C H A P T E R   3 9

Disorders of Elimination

Select the single best response for each question.

39.1   Which of the following statements regarding the clinical presentation of enuresis is *true*?

    A. About 80% of patients with enuresis have primary enuresis.

    B. Without treatment, the remission rate is 30%–50% per year, which decreases with age.

    C. Enuresis continues into adulthood in approximately 8% of cases.

    D. There is no identified increase prevalence of emotional–behavioral disorders in the enuretic population, when compared to the general population.

    E. Clear association between enuresis and tic disorders has been demonstrated.

39.2   Which of the following circumstances would be consistent with a child meeting DSM-IV-TR (American Psychiatric Association 2000) diagnostic criteria for enuresis?

    A. The child must be at least 3 years of age and demonstrate repeated voiding of urine in his or her bed or clothes at least twice weekly for 3 consecutive months.

    B. The child must be at least 3 years of age and demonstrate repeated voiding of urine in his or her bed or clothes at least five times weekly for 6 consecutive months.

    C. The child must be at least 3 years of age and demonstrate repeated voiding of urine in his or her bed or clothes that is not due to a physiological condition.

    D. The child must be at least 5 years of age and demonstrate repeated voiding of urine in his or her bed or clothes at least twice weekly for 3 consecutive months.

    E. The child must be at least 5 years of age and demonstrate repeated voiding of urine in his or her bed or clothes at least five times weekly for 6 consecutive months.

39.3   All of the following statements regarding treatment of enuresis are correct *except*

    A. Enuresis is largely a self-limited, benign disorder.

    B. It is important to provide reassurance support to prevent secondary emotional effects.

    C. Treatment should be preceded by a period of observation and tracking of symptoms.

    D. The most effective treatment for primary enuresis is the enuresis alarm.

    E. Pharmacological interventions include desmopressin (DDAVP), imipramine, and methylphenidate.

39.4   Which of the following statements regarding encopresis is *true*?

    A. Primary encopresis is not preceded by a period of fecal continence.

    B. Secondary encopresis may account for 10%–20% of all cases.

    C. Encopresis resulting from constipation and overflow incontinence is a rare form of the disorder.

    D. Children with encopresis characterized by intentional depositing or smearing of feces are less likely to demonstrate defiant behaviors than are children with encopresis with overflow incontinence.

    E. Most children with functional encopresis demonstrate severe behavioral problems.

39.5 Which of the following statements regarding the treatment of encopresis is *true?*

A. Treatment typically includes medical interventions alone.
B. Treatment requires little evaluation because of the ease with which encopresis is diagnosed.
C. Treatment in children who retain feces should include education, disimpaction, and bowel training.
D. Treatment should not include aversive consequences for soiling accidents.
E. Biofeedback appears to be the most effective available treatment.

C H A P T E R   4 0

Somatoform Disorders

Select the single best response for each question.

40.1 A useful construct, for the purpose of clinical practice, is the separation of illness into five phases. Which of the following represents the correct sequence of these phases?

 A. Vulnerability to disease, adaptation or reaction to the illness, symptom onset, recurrence, chronicity of the disease state.
 B. Vulnerability to disease, symptom onset, recurrence, chronicity of the disease state, adaptation or reaction to the illness.
 C. Vulnerability to disease, adaptation or reaction to the illness, chronicity of the disease state, symptom onset, recurrence.
 D. Adaptation or reaction to the illness, vulnerability to disease, symptom onset, recurrence, chronicity of the disease state.
 E. Adaptation or reaction to the illness, vulnerability to disease, chronicity of the disease state, symptom onset, recurrence.

40.2 For the child psychiatrist attempting to assess the contribution of psychosocial factors to a particular patient's symptoms or illness, several key principles should be kept in mind. Which of the following is *not* one of these key principles?

 A. A significant psychosomatic element is possible in every disorder.
 B. A lack of satisfying findings on physical examination is adequate evidence for ascribing a psychological explanation to a specific case.
 C. Even in diseases in which psychosocial factors have been widely recognized, it is possible for the psychological components to be only minimally important for a particular child's illness.
 D. A lack of typical major psychopathology diagnosable in either the child or the family does not preclude the possibility that psychological factors are influencing the illness to a significant degree.
 E. Psychiatric examination should identify a combination of intrapsychic and environmental factors of sufficient magnitude and likelihood to affect the course of the disorder before psychosocial intervention is undertaken.

40.3 Which of the following statements concerning the psychological evaluation of a child with a physical illness is *false*?

 A. Especially important in the history is a chronology of the relationship between physical symptoms and emotional or stressful periods.
 B. Standard psychological assessment instruments are particularly useful with children who are physically ill.
 C. Having the child or parents keep a journal in which daily entries track important variables can be an asset in understanding a complicated picture.
 D. Physiological measures can be helpful in the psychosomatic assessment of specific children.
 E. None of the above.

40.4 Which of the following would *not* be an appropriate guideline for clinicians working with families who resist psychiatric evaluation?

    A. Establish a final etiological diagnosis.

    B. Concentrate on the psychosocial history, common sources of stress, family psychiatric history, and emotional consequences of the dysfunction.

    C. Suggest focusing on the dysfunction rather than on a diagnosis.

    D. Advocate patience, with the hope that time will foster a sufficient relationship.

    E. Suggest an "if–then" approach, encouraging the family to agree in advance to accept a referral if the last round of diagnostic test results are negative.

40.5 Which of the following would *not* be an appropriate guideline for a clinician initiating therapy with a chronically ill child and his or her family?

    A. The therapist must respect the reality of the medical situation.

    B. The therapist must confront the family's somatic disposition early in therapy, encouraging them to think and speak in psychological, not somatic, terms.

    C. The therapist must respect the patient's creativity in discovering coping solutions.

    D. The therapist must bear in mind that the standards used for judging mental health, defenses, and developmental progression in physically healthy children often do not apply or are only partially relevant to children with chronic illness.

    E. The therapist must refrain from underestimating or minimizing the stressors associated with having a chronic or potentially fatal illness.

C H A P T E R 4 1

Adjustment and Reactive Disorders

Select the single best response for each question.

41.1 The diagnosis of adjustment disorder in children and adolescents

A. Has a focus similar to that in other psychiatric disorders, emphasizing observable symptoms and internalized experiences as primary components of the condition.

B. Elevates the importance of families and outside systems because of its emphasis on psychosocial stressors.

C. Requires that symptoms develop within 6 months of the onset of the stressors.

D. Requires that the presenting symptoms be similar to what would be expected for any child exposed to the stressor in question.

E. Is warranted when symptoms continue for years after the termination of the stressor.

41.2 Which of the following statements regarding cultural syndromes and issues affecting child and adolescent patients is *true*?

A. Cultural syndromes are considered pathological conditions.

B. Cultural syndromes may be best understood by obtaining collateral information from family members or others knowledgeable about the individual's culture.

C. Changes in functioning that do not exceed the bounds of culturally sanctioned phenomena are likely to have long-term negative sequelae.

D. In a study by Bird et al. (1989), the authors reported the culturally specific finding that Puerto Rican children in single-parent families had higher rates of childhood psychopathology than did U.S. mainland children in single-parent families.

E. Bird et al. (1989) suggested that the prominent role played by extended families in the U.S. likely was protective for these children.

41.3 All of the following factors can likely amplify the impact of an identifiable stressor on a child *except*

A. Cognitive immaturity.

B. Preexisting low self-esteem.

C. More primitive defense mechanisms.

D. More accurate understanding of cause-and-effect relationships.

E. Treatment side effects.

41.4 In Kovacs et al.'s (1994) controlled prospective study of children with adjustment disorder, which of the following findings was reported?

A. More than half of the study group children reported a history of suicidal ideation after the onset of the stressor.
B. More than half of the study population had suffered the death of a parent.
C. The median time to recovery after symptom onset was 3 months.
D. Close to 100% recovery was reported in the study population within 12 months.
E. The study group evidenced significantly more long-term sequelae compared with the control group.

41.5 In Kovacs et al.'s (1995) study of children hospitalized for acute-onset diabetes, all of the following findings were reported *except*

A. Seventy-three percent of adjustment disorder diagnoses were made during the first month after the diabetes diagnosis.
B. The first month posthospitalization was the period of greatest psychological vulnerability.
C. Greater vulnerability during the first month postdiagnosis may be related to physiological factors.
D. Short-term psychiatric outcomes for the study population were poor.
E. The presence of adjustment disorder was a risk factor for developing other psychiatric illnesses within the next 5 years.

C H A P T E R   4 2

Personality Disorders

Select the single best response for each question.

42.1   In DSM-IV-TR (American Psychiatric Association 2000), personality disorder categories may be applied to children and adolescents if which of the following criteria is satisfied?

A. The maladaptive personality traits appear to be pervasive and persistent.
B. The maladaptive personality traits appeared before age 12 years.
C. The maladaptive personality traits have been present for at least 6 months.
D. The maladaptive traits appeared before age 7 years.
E. None of the above.

42.2   The New York Longitudinal Study (Thomas and Chess 1977) showed that between the ages of 3 months and 2 years, the *least* stable personality characteristic was

A. Mood.
B. Activity level.
C. Adaptability.
D. Approach behavior.
E. Intensity.

42.3   In DSM-IV-TR, personality disorders are grouped into clusters. Into which cluster do avoidant, dependent, and obsessive-compulsive personality disorders fall?

A. Cluster A.
B. Cluster B.
C. Cluster C.
D. Cluster D.
E. None of the above.

42.4   Diagnostic criteria for histrionic personality disorder include all of the following *except*

A. Is uncomfortable in situations in which he or she is not the center of attention.
B. Displays rapidly shifting and shallow expression of emotions.
C. Shows self-dramatization.
D. Experiences chronic feelings of emptiness.
E. Is suggestible.

42.5   Children with borderline personality disorder commonly

A. Report kinesthetic and tactile hallucinations.
B. Play in an age-appropriate manner.
C. Exhibit empathy for others.
D. Have surprisingly good relationships with peers.
E. Play in a compulsive fashion, without evidence of enjoyment.

CHAPTER 43

Substance Abuse Disorders

Select the single best response for each question.

43.1   Which of the following has been reported to be a problem in applying DSM-IV-TR (American Psychiatric Association 2000) criteria to adolescents?

    A. Withdrawal and drug-related medical problems are common.
    B. One abuse symptom yields a diagnosis.
    C. Abuse symptoms frequently precede dependence symptoms.
    D. Two dependence symptoms with no abuse symptoms yields a diagnosis.
    E. None of the above.

43.2   In the 2001 Monitoring the Future Survey (Johnston et al. 2001), epidemiological findings concerning substance abuse in high school seniors included all of the following *except*

    A. Marijuana use by about 37%.
    B. Cigarette smoking during the past month by 29.5%.
    C. MDMA (3,4-methylenedioxymethamphetamine; "ecstasy") use by 9.2%.
    D. Anabolic steroid use by 12.4%.
    E. Alcohol use by about 73%.

43.3   The well-known CAGE screening questions developed for adults are not useful for adolescents. The CRAFFT, a screening instrument developed for adolescents, includes all of the following questions *except*

    A. "Have you ever ridden in a **C**ar driven by someone (including yourself) who was high or had been using alcohol or drugs?"
    B. "Do you ever use alcohol/drugs to **R**elax, feel better about yourself, or fit in?"
    C. "Do you get **A**ngry when you are told that you have a problem?"
    D. "Do you ever **F**orget things you did while using alcohol/drugs?"
    E. "Have you ever gotten into **T**rouble while you were using alcohol/drugs?"

43.4   Risk factors for the development of substance abuse disorders include all of the following *except*

    A. Economic and social advantage.
    B. School failure.
    C. Friends who use drugs.
    D. Psychiatric comorbidity.
    E. History of parental divorce.

43.5 A common comorbid diagnosis in male adolescents with substance abuse is

  A. Conduct disorder.
  B. Attention-deficit/hyperactivity disorder.
  C. Avoidant personality disorder.
  D. Oppositional defiant disorder.
  E. None of the above.

C H A P T E R 4 4

Gender Identity and Psychosexual Disorders

Select the single best response for each question.

44.1 Which of the following statements concerning gender identity is *false?*

A. Gender identity typically appears in its nascent form between 2 and 3 years of age.
B. Children 2–3 years of age are able to categorize people by sex on the basis of phenotypic social cues, such as clothing or hairstyle.
C. *Gender identity* refers to a person's behavioral adoption of cultural markers of masculinity and femininity.
D. The ability to categorize others by sex likely precedes the ability to self-categorize oneself as a boy or girl.
E. None of the above.

44.2 In children, according to DSM-IV-TR (American Psychiatric Association 2000), gender identity disorder is manifested by which of the following?

A. A repeatedly stated desire to be, or insistence that he or she is, the other sex.
B. Strong and persistent preferences for cross-sex roles in make-believe play.
C. An intense desire to participate in the stereotypical games and pastimes of the other sex.
D. A strong preference for playmates of the other sex.
E. All of the above.

44.3 The age at onset of cross-gender behavior in gender identity disorder is typically

A. Before the age of 5 years.
B. Between the ages of 6 and 10 years.
C. Between the ages of 12 and 15 years.
D. Between the ages of 16 and 19 years.
E. None of the above.

44.4 Which of the following statements concerning biophysical markers in children with gender identity disorder is *true?*

A. Standard endocrine assessments frequently detect abnormalities.
B. Abnormal XY karyotypes have been reported in boys.
C. Feminine boys are shorter and weigh less than nonfeminine boys at the time of assessment.
D. All of the above.
E. None of the above.

44.5 Scholars who have reworked the original Kinsey report concerning the prevalence of homosexuality in men (Kinsey et al. 1948) estimate rates in the range of

A. 1%–2%.
B. 2%–6%.
C. 6%–10%.
D. 10%–12%.
E. None of the above.

CHAPTER 45

Physical Abuse of Children

Select the single best response for each question.

45.1 Which of the following statements concerning the epidemiology of physical abuse of children is *false*?

A. Younger children (less than 3 years of age) have the greatest risk of fatal maltreatment.
B. Homicides occurring during the first week of life are almost exclusively perpetrated by mothers.
C. Fathers are more likely to fatally injure their children ages 1 week to 13 years.
D. Fathers committed the majority of parent-perpetrated homicides of children 13–19 years of age.
E. None of the above.

45.2 Risk factors that may predict recurrence of abuse in children include which of the following?

A. Young age of the child.
B. Number of previous referrals to child protective services.
C. History of childhood abuse in the caretaker.
D. Prematurity, mental retardation, or physical handicaps in the child.
E. All of the above.

45.3 Indicators suggesting possible physical abuse in a child who presents with an injury include all of the following *except*

A. Observation of an inappropriate history for the injury.
B. A reasonable explanation for the injury.
C. An excessive or inadequate level of concern in the parent.
D. Delay in seeking medical attention.
E. A contradictory, changing, or vague history of the injury.

45.4 Which of the following characteristics in children should increase a clinician's suspicion of possible physical abuse?

A. A child who is afraid to leave home.
B. A child who craves physical contact.
C. A child with excessive needs for being comforted.
D. A child who is on the alert for danger.
E. All of the above.

45.5 Physical findings in an injured child suggestive of physical abuse include which of the following?

A. Bruises or lacerations in the shape of an object.
B. Posterior rib fractures.
C. Anogenital lacerations.
D. Twisting injuries of the ear lobe.
E. All of the above.

CHAPTER 46

Sexual Abuse of Children

Select the single best response for each question.

46.1　Which of the following statements concerning sexual abuse of boys is *false?*

A. Perpetrators of abuse against boys are most likely to be related to the victim.
B. Boys are less likely than girls to disclose abuse.
C. Surveys indicate that as many as 18% of males older than 18 years report having been victims of childhood sexual abuse.
D. Perpetrators of abuse against boys are most likely to be male.
E. Sexual abuse of boys may be significantly underreported and untreated.

46.2　In comparison with the general population, persons who perpetrate sexual abuse

A. Are more frequently from lower socioeconomic classes.
B. Are less likely to have been raised in families with a history of domestic violence.
C. Are more likely to have been abused as children.
D. Are less likely to be practicing a religion.
E. Are more often of minority race/ethnicity.

46.3　Perpetrators of sexual abuse

A. Are often children and adolescents.
B. Are gender specific regarding their choice of victims.
C. Often associate themselves with events or activities in which they have access to children.
D. May seek to "groom" victims with gifts or money.
E. All of the above.

46.4　Psychiatric disorders often found in sexually abused children include all of the following *except*

A. Depression.
B. Bipolar disorder.
C. Anxiety disorders.
D. Schizophrenia.
E. Eating disorders.

46.5　Key points to consider when conducting a forensic evaluation of a child for suspected sexual abuse include all of the following *except*

A. A stepwise interview approach, starting with nonabuse topics and progressing to abuse topics, works best.
B. Psychological testing and screening checklists may provide definitive evidence of abuse.
C. A gentle, nonthreatening demeanor that avoids retraumatization is essential.
D. Biased or leading questions should be avoided.
E. Specialized techniques, such as the use of drawings or anatomical dolls, may be useful for younger children but are not essential.

CHAPTER 47

HIV and AIDS: Global and United States Perspectives

Select the single best response for each question.

47.1   All of the following statistics concerning human immunodeficiency virus (HIV)/acquired immunodeficiency syndrome (AIDS) worldwide in 2002 are correct *except*

   A. 3.2 million children younger than 15 years of age were living with HIV/AIDS.
   B. 800,000 children became newly infected with HIV.
   C. Less than 100,000 children younger than 15 years of age died of AIDS.
   D. 19.2 million women were infected with HIV/AIDS.
   E. 1.2 million women died of AIDS.

47.2   As of June 2001, the most common exposure group for U.S. children younger than 13 years of age with AIDS was

   A. Children born to mothers who are injection drug users or sexual partners of HIV-infected males.
   B. Children with hemophilia or coagulation disorder.
   C. Recipients of transfusion, blood components, or tissue.
   D. Undetermined.
   E. None of the above.

47.3   Which of the following is the preferred method for diagnosing HIV in infancy?

   A. HIV RNA assay in plasma.
   B. HIV culture.
   C. DNA polymerase chain reaction (PCR) assay.
   D. Presence of maternal antibodies.
   E. Enzyme-linked immunosorbent assay (ELISA).

47.4   As of June 2001, the *least* common exposure route for U.S. adolescents between the ages of 13 and 19 years with AIDS was

   A. High-risk sexual contact.
   B. Injection drug use.
   C. Blood transfusion or coagulation disorder.
   D. Undetermined.
   E. None of the above.

47.5 According to guidelines of the American Academy of Child and Adolescent Psychiatry (1995), HIV-infected adolescents who require inpatient psychiatric or substance abuse treatment

A. Should be denied admission.
B. Should be segregated from other patients.
C. Should be assigned to individual rooms.
D. Should be treated with universal precautionary measures, unlike HIV-negative patients.
E. None of the above.

C H A P T E R   4 8
Suicide and Suicidality

Select the single best response for each question.

48.1 Self-mutilation

    A. Is defined as superficial cutting of the arms, legs, and other body areas.

    B. Is rarely associated with stress.

    C. Always involves a clear intention to kill oneself.

    D. Is never associated with suicidal intent.

    E. Is rarely associated with dissociative phenomena.

48.2 Which of the following statements concerning epidemiological findings in youth suicide is *false*?

    A. Suicide among black youth has increased more rapidly than that among white youth.

    B. Increased rates of youth suicide are associated with greater availability of firearms.

    C. Male youths are more likely to attempt suicide than are females.

    D. Approximately 1% of preadolescents in the general population report having made a suicide attempt.

    E. None of the above.

48.3 Which of the following childhood environmental stressors has been identified as a suicide risk factor?

    A. Adolescent unemployment.

    B. Family history of suicidal behavior.

    C. Poor communication with the mother or the father.

    D. Adolescent suspension from school.

    E. All of the above.

48.4 A "psychological autopsy" study of 67 adolescent suicide victims found greatly elevated risks for suicide associated with certain psychiatric disorders (Brent et al. 1993). Which of the following disorders imparted the greatest increase in risk?

    A. Attention-deficit/hyperactivity disorder.

    B. Alcohol abuse.

    C. Schizophrenia.

    D. Major depression.

    E. Conduct disorder.

48.5 Research studies examining treatment targeted toward prevention of child and adolescent suicide have reported which of the following findings?

    A. Unlike the case in adults, depression is not a key risk factor for suicide in children and adolescents.

    B. Utilization of mental health treatment among depressed youths is high, approaching 75%.

    C. Presence or absence of health insurance coverage has little to do with whether children receive antidepressant treatment.

    D. Family functioning typically has little association with suicidal behavior in youths.

    E. Children and adolescents who attempt suicide are often first evaluated in emergency departments.

CHAPTER 49

Forensic Psychiatry

Select the single best response for each question.

49.1 The White House Conference on Children, convened in 1970 (U.S. Government Printing Office 1971), asserted all of the following specific rights as central to a child's well-being *except*

A. The right to be born and to be healthy and wanted throughout childhood.
B. The right to mental health care, regardless of socioeconomic status.
C. The right to be educated to the limits of one's capability.
D. The right to grow up nurtured by affectionate parents.
E. The right to have societal mechanisms to enforce the foregoing rights.

49.2 Which of the following standards of proof is required in juvenile court and delinquency proceedings?

A. Reasonable degree of certainty.
B. Clear and convincing evidence.
C. Beyond a reasonable doubt.
D. Preponderance of the evidence.
E. More likely than not.

49.3 Special ethical dimensions that distinguish the care and treatment of children include which of the following?

A. The child is a minor, and parental involvement is necessary to some degree.
B. The child's developmental maturation expands the capacity for understanding and judgment and responsibility for behavior.
C. The child is involved with school and perhaps other social agencies and institutions that require exchange of information and collaboration in the care and treatment efforts.
D. All of the above.
E. None of the above.

49.4 Which of the following is *not* an element of informed consent?

A. The clinician must inform the patient of the nature of the condition and the recommended treatment, including benefits and risks.
B. The clinician must adhere to the professional practice standard prevailing at the time in the community.
C. The patient's choice must be voluntary.
D. The patient must have the capacity to consent.
E. The clinician should inform the patient of alternatives to the recommended treatment, including their risks and benefits.

49.5 The essential elements of professional malpractice include all of the following *except*

    A. A duty of care was owed to the patient by the physician.
    B. The proper diagnosis was not made.
    C. The patient experienced actual damage due to the breach of duty.
    D. The duty of care was breached.
    E. The dereliction was the direct cause of the damages.

49.6 The current guiding principle in deciding child custody disputes is

    A. The wishes of the parent.
    B. The mental and physical health of the parents.
    C. The interactions of the child with those who may significantly affect his or her best interests.
    D. The wishes of the child.
    E. The best interests of the child.

C H A P T E R   5 0

Psychopharmacology

Select the single best response for each question.

50.1 Commonly reported and well-substantiated side effects of stimulant medications include all of the following *except*

    A. Appetite suppression.
    B. Sleep disturbance.
    C. Mild increases in pulse and blood pressure.
    D. Stunting of growth in height.
    E. Weight loss.

50.2 A number of studies have evaluated the short- and long-term effects of therapeutic doses of tricyclic antidepressants (TCAs) on the cardiovascular system in children. Which of the following statements is *incorrect?*

    A. TCAs are generally well tolerated.
    B. TCAs may produce electrocardiographic abnormalities at doses between 1 and 2 mg/kg.
    C. Patients should be carefully monitored at higher TCA doses (greater than 3.5 mg/kg).
    D. Before initiating TCAs, a baseline electrocardiogram is recommended.
    E. None of the above.

50.3 Some compounds metabolized by the cytochrome P450 enzyme 3A4 have been associated with QT prolongations when combined with drugs that inhibit 3A4. Antidepressants that affect 3A4 activity include all of the following *except*

    A. Fluvoxamine.
    B. Venlafaxine.
    C. Nefazodone.
    D. Fluoxetine.
    E. Sertraline.

50.4 Novel atypical antipsychotic medications exert their therapeutic effects through antagonism of which of the following receptors?

    A. Dopaminergic (D_1).
    B. Histaminic (H_1).
    C. Serotonergic ($5\text{-}HT_2$).
    D. Alpha$_1$-adrenergic.
    E. None of the above.

50.5 Oxcarbazepine is chemically similar to carbamazepine with some important differences, which include all of the following *except*

A. Laboratory monitoring is still required with oxcarbazepine.
B. Oxcarbazepine has little interaction with the cytochrome P450 system.
C. Oxcarbazepine lacks the hepatic liability of carbamazepine.
D. Oxcarbazepine does not induce its own metabolism.
E. Oxcarbazepine lacks the hematological liability of carbamazepine.

50.6 In child psychiatry, clonidine is commonly used in the treatment of all of the following *except*

A. Attention-deficit/hyperactivity disorder (ADHD).
B. Tourette's disorder.
C. Aggression.
D. Sleep disturbance in ADHD children.
E. Major depressive disorder.

50.7 Side effects associated with the use of atomoxetine in children include which of the following?

A. Increased appetite.
B. Cardiac conduction delays.
C. Insomnia.
D. Increase in pulse and diastolic blood pressure.
E. Abuse.

C H A P T E R   5 1

Psychoanalysis and Psychodynamic Therapy

Select the single best response for each question.

51.1 Melanie Klein's technique of child psychoanalysis is based on which of the following fundamental principles?

A. Verbalization and clarification of the preconscious material.
B. Suggestions and educational efforts.
C. Play as the child's mode of free association.
D. Reassuring of the child as part of a trusting relationship with an adult.
E. All of the above.

51.2 Although Anna Freud's system of child psychoanalysis was based on the traditional adult model, she recognized that children in analysis differ from adult analysands in which of the following ways?

A. Children do not seek out therapy on their own.
B. Children may have little motivation for cure.
C. Children tend to deny problems and try to externalize their causes rather than accept responsibility for them.
D. Children will run away from discomfort and so will not easily relinquish fantasy for reality.
E. All of the above.

51.3 In psychodynamic psychotherapy with children, in contrast to child psychoanalysis,

A. Children are not usually seen 5 days per week.
B. Corrective emotional experiences are encouraged rather than viewed as obstacles to self-awareness.
C. The parents are often greatly involved in treatment.
D. Children are given more active support and practical guidance.
E. All of the above.

51.4 In regard to how play is conceptualized in psychodynamic psychotherapy, all of the following statements are correct *except*

A. Play is taken as the child's description of his or her perception of the universe.
B. Play is used as a substitute for free association.
C. Children project their inner lives into their play activity.
D. Play is used as a child's mode for communicating the totality of his or her current life.
E. Play allows the child to present his or her predicament "in displacement," as if it did not specifically pertain to the child.

51.5   Evaluating the effectiveness of psychotherapy with children or adolescents is difficult, because a number of factors besides the clinical needs of patients can substantially affect the results. In evaluating study reports of therapeutic effectiveness, which of the following potential influences should be considered?

A. The relative dysfunction of the child's family or environment.
B. The developmental level of the child.
C. The compliance of the parents with therapy recommendations.
D. The extent of treatment goals.
E. All of the above.

C H A P T E R   5 2

Cognitive-Behavior Modification

Select the single best response for each question.

52.1 Behavior modification is based largely on two conceptual views of affect, cognition, and behavior: mediational and nonmediational. Which of the following statements describes the *mediational view?*

   A. It focuses on direct connections between environmental or situational events and behaviors.
   B. It emphasizes constructs such as affect and cognition that underlie behavior.
   C. It is the basis for operant conditioning.
   D. It conceptualizes child problems as deficits or excesses in performance.
   E. None of the above.

52.2 Cognitive-behavioral therapy for anxiety in children focuses on dysfunctional cognitions and their implications for the child's subsequent thinking and behavior. The term *cognitive distortions* refers to

   A. Attributions that result from cognitive structures, content, and processes.
   B. How experiences are processed and interpreted.
   C. Information processes that lead to misperceptions of oneself or the environment.
   D. Memory and ways in which information is experienced.
   E. None of the above.

52.3 *Consequential thinking*, an example of a cognitive problem-solving skill, is defined as

   A. The ability to identify what might happen as a direct result of acting in a particular way.
   B. The ability to relate one event to another over time and to understand why one event led to a particular action.
   C. The ability to perceive a problem when it exists and to identify the interpersonal aspects of the confrontation that may emerge.
   D. The ability to generate different options that can solve problems.
   E. The ability to be aware of the intermediate steps required to achieve a particular goal.

52.4 Parent management training (PMT) is one of the best-researched therapy techniques for children and adolescents. Which of the following statements concerning PMT is *false?*

   A. PMT is quite effective in treating conduct disorder.
   B. PMT has led to marked improvements in child behavior, as reflected in parent and teacher reports of deviant behavior.
   C. Children and adolescents with conduct behavior problems who have been treated with PMT have achieved normative levels of functioning at home and at school.
   D. Treatment gains for children treated with PMT are short-lived (less than 6 months).
   E. None of the above.

52.5 Punishment procedures employed in operant conditioning treatments include which of the following?

A. Time-out from reinforcement.
B. Applying response cost.
C. Overcorrection.
D. All of the above.
E. None of the above.

CHAPTER 53
Family Therapy

Select the single best response for each question.

53.1   Which of the following is *not* a goal of the psychotherapeutic modality *family therapy*?

   A. Exploring the interactional dynamics of the family and their relation to psychopathology.
   B. Identifying psychopathology in individual family members and referring them for treatment.
   C. Mobilizing the family's internal strengths and functional resources.
   D. Restructuring maladaptive interactional family styles.
   E. Strengthening the family's problem-solving behavior.

53.2   Which of the following family therapy investigators developed the concept of the *undifferentiation phenomenon* and its relation to the transmission of anxiety within the family system?

   A. Bowen.
   B. Bateson.
   C. Satir.
   D. Minuchin.
   E. Haley.

53.3   Different models of family therapy are applicable to different patient populations. Which of the following models is specifically applicable to seriously and chronically disabled families with concomitant disintegration in the family and its social network?

   A. Structural and strategic family therapy.
   B. Behavioral family therapy.
   C. Intergenerational family therapy.
   D. Psychodynamic and experiential family therapy.
   E. Social network therapy.

53.4   The theoretical concept of the *boundary* forms the foundation of which of the following types of family therapy?

   A. Contextual therapy.
   B. Experiential family therapy.
   C. Behavioral family therapy.
   D. Structural family therapy.
   E. Psychodynamic family therapy.

53.5   The rate of relapse among schizophrenic and depressed patients has been reported to be much higher in some families than in others. What family variable has been found to be closely linked to these high relapse rates?

   A. No expressed emotion.
   B. Low expressed emotion.
   C. High expressed emotion.
   D. High cognitive orientation.
   E. Low cognitive orientation.

C H A P T E R 5 4

Group Psychotherapy

Select the single best response for each question.

54.1 Which of the following categories of adolescent therapy groups does *not* require a therapeutic contract?

A. Para-analytic psychotherapy groups.
B. Therapeutic groups.
C. Educational and sensitivity groups.
D. Self-help groups.
E. Multifamily groups.

54.2 Which of the following statements concerning cognitive-behavior therapy (CBT) groups is *false*?

A. They can be adapted for all age groups.
B. They may be used in a variety of settings.
C. They may be used to treat a variety of presenting problems.
D. They are generally long-term and not skills-specific.
E. In these groups, the child is expected to be an active participant.

54.3 Group play therapy

A. Is usually conducted in a large playroom setting.
B. Uses simple and generic play materials.
C. Generally involves weekly meetings.
D. Will vary in length depending on the developmental level of the child.
E. All of the above.

54.4 After initial startup tasks, expressive and art therapy group sessions for older children and adolescents consist of four phases. Which of the following is *not* a phase of this modality?

A. Motivation (warm-up).
B. Closure.
C. The art activity.
D. Evaluation of the child's art ability.
E. Discussion of the process and product (sharing).

54.5 Which of the following is a type of self-help group?

A. Permanent group.
B. Addiction group.
C. Crisis group.
D. All of the above.
E. None of the above.

C H A P T E R   5 5

Hypnosis

Select the single best response for each question.

55.1   An understanding of hypnosis emphasizes the essential features of absorption, dissociation, and suggestibility. *Absorption* is defined as

A. The relative suspension of peripheral awareness.
B. The tendency to accept instruction uncritically.
C. A receptive, trusting rapport.
D. The characteristic state of attentive, receptive focal concentration.
E. None of the above.

55.2   The Hypnotic Induction Profile (HIP; Spiegel and Spiegel 1978) measures and correlates the subject's patterns of responses to instructions for

A. Eye roll.
B. Dissociation.
C. Posthypnotic arm levitation.
D. Posthypnotic subjective experiences.
E. All of the above.

55.3   The greater hypnotizability of children compared with adults is believed to be due to all of the following factors *except*

A. Emotional malleability.
B. Broader cognitive focus.
C. Openness to new experiences.
D. Intrinsic orientation to learning new skills.
E. Ease in accepting regressive phenomena.

55.4   Hypnosis has been used to treat a wide array of psychiatric and medical disorders in children and adolescents. Which of the following disorders is the best-established and most systematically studied indication for hypnosis?

A. Pain.
B. Seizure disorders.
C. Anxiety disorders.
D. Gastrointestinal disorders.
E. Dissociative identity disorder.

55.5   Hypnosis is generally *not* appropriate for which of the following mental disorders?

A. Dissociative identity disorder.
B. Anxiety disorders.
C. Childhood habit disorders.
D. Trichotillomania.
E. Psychotic disorders.

CHAPTER 56

Milieu Therapy:
Inpatient, Partial, Residential

Select the single best response for each question.

56.1 Critical psychological factors for psychiatrists to consider when admitting or discharging children and adolescents who represent a potential danger to themselves or others include the presence of

    A. Persecutory delusions.
    B. Command hallucinations.
    C. Paranoia.
    D. Impaired executive functioning that would take into account the presence of alcohol or substance abuse.
    E. All of the above.

56.2 Critical elements of a master treatment plan include all of the following *except*

    A. Psychiatric symptoms.
    B. Insurance coverage.
    C. Medical issues.
    D. Discharge.
    E. Psychoeducation.

56.3 Which of the following factors differentiates a residential treatment center (RTC) from a psychiatric inpatient unit?

    A. Individuals staying in an RTC perceive themselves as residents rather than as patients.
    B. Meeting of dependency needs is paramount in an RTC.
    C. More regression is expected in an RTC.
    D. All of the above.
    E. None of the above.

56.4 The focus of inpatient care currently includes all of the following *except*

    A. Transition to less restrictive settings.
    B. Stabilization.
    C. Medical treatment.
    D. Disposition planning.
    E. Assessment.

56.5 Broadly defined, *day treatment* refers to which of the following?

    A. School-based care.
    B. Care provided for at least 5 hours per day.
    C. Integrated education, counseling, and family services.
    D. All of the above.
    E. None of the above.

C H A P T E R   1

Development of the Subspecialty of Child and Adolescent Psychiatry in the United States

Select the single best response for each question.

1.1 The initial purposes of the Academy of Child Psychiatry included all of the following *except*

A. Delineate the scope of the specialty and its practice.
B. Set standards of training and practice.
C. Stimulate physicians to enter the field of child psychiatry.
D. Enroll all practicing child psychiatrists.
E. Promote and advance prevention, treatment, research, and teaching in the field.

The correct response is option D.

The initial purposes of the Academy of Child Psychiatry were to define the scope and standards of the field, to stimulate interest in the field, and to advance practice and training. Membership was by invitation only and required 5 years of practice in the field. The Academy became a general membership organization in 1969. **(p. 4)**

1.2 Erik Erikson's classic text *Childhood and Society* (1950) emphasized the principles of which of the following as important for understanding normal development and psychopathology in childhood?

A. Psychoanalysis.
B. Ego psychology.
C. Family therapy.
D. Behavior therapy.
E. Crisis intervention.

The correct response is option B.

Many different theoretical perspectives have shaped the understanding of development and of psychopathology in childhood. These perspectives include psychoanalysis, family therapy, behavior therapy, and others. Erikson's (1950) text emphasized the principles of ego psychology, introduced by Anna Freud (1946), highlighting the interplay between intrapsychic and environmental variables. **(p. 6)**

1.3   Szurek (1942) and Johnson (1949) used the term *superego lacunae* to describe which of the following?

A. Neuronal abnormalities in cortical development of delinquents.
B. Gaps in family structure (parental absence) in the families of delinquent adolescents.
C. Positive magnetic resonance imaging findings suggesting basal ganglia pathology in delinquents.
D. Developmental abnormalities in the language functioning of delinquents.
E. The contribution of unconscious parental permission to the antisocial acts of delinquents.

The correct response is option E.

The term *superego lacunae* was introduced to describe how parents may unconsciously give signals to their children that certain delinquent acts are permissible. The term does not refer to neurological abnormalities or deficits of family structure, both of which can also contribute to delinquency. **(p. 7)**

1.4   Which of the following researchers focused on the important contributions of temperament to child development?

A. Chess and Thomas.
B. Bowlby.
C. Piaget.
D. Spitz.
E. Brazelton.

The correct response is option A.

Chess et al. (1963) and Thomas et al. (1968) conducted pioneering research in which they prospectively followed a cohort of children, examining the impact of temperament on their development. Bowlby's (1969, 1973) contributions were in the areas of attachment and loss. Piaget (1926) focused on cognitive development. Spitz (1945, 1946) emphasized the developmental impact of early maternal loss and deprivation. Brazelton et al. (1966) recognized the early competencies of infants in influencing the mother–infant relationship. **(p. 8)**

1.5   Which of the following statements about managed care and its impact on child psychiatry is *false*?

A. Managed care was designed to contain the rising costs of health care.
B. Managed care may limit the ability of child psychiatrists to provide adequate care to patients.
C. Managed care decisions related to treatments of choice are based on well-documented and well-conducted outcome studies.
D. Managed care may require child psychiatrists to serve in an advocacy role for their patients.
E. Managed care decisions may be driven more by cost considerations than by treatment considerations.

The correct response is option C.

Managed care was designed to limit the escalation in national health care spending. A potential consequence of managed care is that cost considerations may negatively influence treatment, limiting available treatment options. In such cases, child psychiatrists may be required to advocate for effective treatments for individual patients. Unfortunately, managed care decisions are not always based on available and well-conducted outcome studies. **(pp. 9–10)**

References

Bowlby J: Attachment and Loss, Vol 1: Attachment. New York, Basic Books, 1969

Bowlby J: Attachment and Loss, Vol 2: Separation, Anxiety, and Anger. London, Hogarth Press, 1973

Brazelton TB, School ML, Robey JF: Visual responses in the newborn. Pediatrics 37:284–290, 1966

Chess S, Thomas A, Rutter M, et al: Interaction of temperament and environment in the production of behavioral disturbances. Am J Psychiatry 120:142–147, 1963

Erikson EH: Childhood and Society. New York, WW Norton, 1950

Freud A: The Ego and the Mechanisms of Defense. New York, International Universities Press, 1946

Johnson A: Sanctions for superego lacunae of adolescents, in Searchlight on Delinquency. Edited by Eissler KR. New York, International Universities Press, 1949, pp 225–245

Piaget J: The Language and Thought of the Child. New York, Harcourt Brace, 1926

Spitz R: Hospitalism: an inquiry into the genesis of psychiatric conditions in early childhood. Psychoanal Study Child 1:53–74, 1945

Spitz R: Anaclitic depression. Psychoanal Study Child 2:313–342, 1946

Szurek SA: Notes on the genesis of psychopathic personality trends. Psychiatry 5:1–6, 1942

Thomas A, Chess S, Birch HG: Temperament and Behavior Disorders in Children. New York, New York University Press, 1968

C H A P T E R 2

Overview of Development From Infancy Through Adolescence

Select the single best response for each question.

2.1   Theories of development formulated by Freud, Erikson, and Piaget share which of the following characteristics?

   A. They postulate a genetically determined capacity for the development of patterns or systems of behavior by the child.
   B. They propose that the overall behavior patterns that emerge are qualitatively similar to one another.
   C. They are all structural theories of development that imply that reorganization within the child is unnecessary.
   D. They postulate that the child reacts in particular ways to environmental stimuli.
   E. None of the above.

The correct response is option A.

Psychoanalysis (Freud), psychosocial development (Erikson), and cognitive development (Piaget), the theories of development known as structural theories, postulate a genetically determined capacity for the development of patterns or systems of behavior in which the child acts on the environment from the beginning. The overall behavior patterns that emerge are qualitatively different from one another but exhibit continuity. Structural theories imply that reorganization within the child is required. Option D characterizes reactive theories, not structural theories. **(p. 16)**

2.2   By age 5 years, a child will have attained all of the following motor developmental milestones *except*

   A. Can stand on one foot.
   B. Can dance and jump.
   C. Manifests firmly established leg, eye, and ear dominance.
   D. Can copy a square.
   E. Can build a tower of 10 cubes.

The correct response is option C.

Leg, eye, and ear dominance may not become firmly established until the seventh, eight, or ninth year of life, respectively. By age 3 years, children can stand on one foot, dance and jump, and build a tower of 10 cubes. At age 5 years, they can copy a square. **(p. 17)**

2.3   Piaget conceptualized four major stages of cognitive development. Which of the following states the correct sequence in which these stages normally occur, from birth to adolescence?

   A. Preoperational, sensorimotor, concrete operational, formal operational.
   B. Concrete operational, sensorimotor, preoperational, formal operational.
   C. Sensorimotor, concrete operational, formal operational, preoperational.
   D. Formal operational, concrete operational, sensorimotor, preoperational.
   E. Sensorimotor, preoperational, concrete operational, formal operational.

The correct response is option E.

Piaget's four major stages of development are sensorimotor (from birth to 2 years), preoperational (from 2 years to 7 years), concrete operational (from 7 years to adolescence), and formal operational (adolescence). **(p. 20)**

2.4   Chunking is

   A. A process by which representations, procedures, and memories that occur together are automatically accessed simultaneously.
   B. A type of long-term memory.
   C. A form of procedural knowledge.
   D. All of the above.
   E. None of the above.

The correct response is option A.

Chunking, which occurs in *short-term memory*, is the process by which representations, procedures, and memories that occur together are automatically accessed simultaneously. *Long-term memory* involves two types of knowledge: declarative knowledge and procedural knowledge. *Declarative knowledge* is knowledge of facts, concepts, and ideas. Amnesia due to brain damage usually results in loss of declarative knowledge. *Procedural knowledge* is knowledge of how to perform certain acts. This kind of knowledge is usually unconscious and is not lost in amnesia due to brain damage. **(pp. 24–25)**

2.5   According to Spitz (1965), organizers that govern the process of transition from one level to the next in the development of attachment include all of the following *except*

   A. Sustained eye contact in response to an interaction.
   B. The smiling response.
   C. Eight-month anxiety.
   D. Achievement of the sign of negation.
   E. None of the above.

The correct response is option A.

Spitz (1965) described three "organizers" in the development of attachment: the smiling response, the 8-month anxiety, and the use of negation and of the word *no*. Spitz did not include sustained eye contact as an organizer. **(p. 30)**

2.6   In psychoanalytic theory, the *anal phase* of psychosexual development is characterized by

A. The child's focus on autoerotic activities.
B. The child's experience of intense sexual and aggressive urges toward both parents.
C. The child's development of concepts of inevitability regarding birth, death, and sex differences.
D. The child's experience of feelings of separateness and worth.
E. The child's sequential development of play.

The correct response is option D.

According to psychoanalytic theory, the four phases of psychosexual development are oral, anal, phallic–oedipal, and latency. During the *anal phase*, the child begins to experience feelings about separateness and worth. The focus on autoerotic activities (self-stimulating) occurs during the *oral phase;* the sequential development of play and intense sexual and aggressive urges occurs during the *phallic–oedipal phase;* and clarification of the inevitability of birth, death, and sex differences occurs during the *latency* phase. **(pp. 31–32)**

Reference

Spitz R: The First Year of Life. New York, International Universities Press, 1965

C H A P T E R   3

Role of Culture, Race, and Ethnicity in Child and Adolescent Psychiatry

Select the single best response for each question.

3.1   Terms such as *race, ethnicity, culture,* and *nationality* are often used synonymously, but each represents a distinct concept. For example, in North America, the term *African American* represents which of the following?

   A. Race and ethnicity.
   B. Race and culture.
   C. Ethnicity and nationality.
   D. Nationality and culture.
   E. None of the above.

The correct response is option E.

African American refers to someone of a black race who was born in the United States (race and nationality); it does *not* refer to all Americans in the United States who identify themselves as being of a black race (e.g., an American of Belizean descent would more likely identify with Central America, not the African continent). *Culture* refers to a broad set of ideas, values, beliefs, and attitudes. *Ethnicity* is one aspect of culture. Although ethnicity refers primarily to *nationality* (i.e., one's citizenship or national identity), it is more specific than culture in that it encompasses group-shared patterns of social interaction and shared values, behaviors, perceptions, and use of language. *Race* is biologically defined, with differentiation generally based on skin color and other physical characteristics. **(p. 45)**

3.2   Cross-cultural psychiatry

   A. Discounts the presence of culture-specific syndromes.
   B. Minimizes the universal applicability of psychiatric diagnoses.
   C. Recognizes that psychiatric conditions may have different characteristics in different cultural and ethnic groups.
   D. Emphasizes the importance of cultural over individual contributions to illness.
   E. Has little clinical research that supports its basic tenets.

The correct response is option C.

Cross-cultural psychiatry is a field of growing interest and importance that is supported by research. It recognizes the importance of cultural contributions in the practice of child and adolescent psychiatry within the context of understanding the individual patient. Cross-cultural psychiatry allows for universal application of psychiatric diagnoses while recognizing that such conditions may present variably in different cultural and ethnic groups. **(pp. 46–47)**

3.3   Konner (1995) described five cross-cultural factors universally present in human development. Which of the following lists the correct developmental order of these factors?

   A. Emergence of socialization, onset of attachments, emergence of language, observable gender-specific aggression, mature sexual motivation.
   B. Onset of attachments, emergence of socialization, observable gender-specific aggression, emergence of language, mature sexual motivation.
   C. Onset of attachments, emergence of language, emergence of socialization, observable gender-specific aggression, mature sexual motivation.
   D. Emergence of language, onset of attachments, emergence of socialization, observable gender-specific aggression, mature sexual motivation.
   E. Emergence of socialization, onset of attachments, observable gender-specific aggression, emergence of language, mature sexual motivation.

The correct response is option A.

The correct sequence of Konner's (1995) cross-cultural universal stages in human development is emergence of socialization (0–4 months), onset of attachments (6–12 months), emergence of language (after 12 months), observable gender-specific physical aggressiveness (early and middle childhood), and mature sexual motivation (adolescence). **(p. 50)**

3.4   Cultural assimilation

   A. Refers to acquiring the norms and values of one's own cultural group.
   B. Is equivalent to biculturalism.
   C. Represents the desire to replace one's own cultural values with those of the host culture.
   D. Allows one to retain significant portions of one's own cultural values while absorbing those of another.
   E. Is correlated with a lower risk of psychopathology in Hispanic adolescents.

The correct response is option C.

Cultural assimilation, one type of acculturation, involves replacing one's own cultural identity and values with that of another. *Acculturation* is defined more flexibly and may also include the process of biculturalism. *Biculturalism* involves taking on characteristics of the host culture while retaining specific aspects of one's own culture. High cultural assimilation has been correlated with a higher, not lower, risk for psychopathology among Hispanic adolescent groups. **(p. 51)**

3.5   All of the following statements about the African American cultural experience in the United States are correct *except*

   A. African Americans constitute the largest minority group in the United States.
   B. African Americans experience higher levels of social, emotional, and financial distress than do whites, regardless of socioeconomic status.
   C. Extended kinship networks provide emotional support for many African American families.
   D. Religious belief and church affiliation provide support to many African Americans.
   E. Stereotypic impressions of African Americans can result in ineffective treatment.

The correct response is option B.

Community surveys have consistently shown that whereas African Americans do, on average, experience higher levels of social, emotional, and financial distress compared with whites, these differences disappear when socioeconomic status is statistically controlled (Canino and Spurlock 2000). **(p. 51)**

References

Canino I, Spurlock J: Culturally Diverse Children and Adolescents: Assessment, Diagnosis and Treatment, 2nd Edition. New York, Guilford, 2000

Konner M: Contributions of the sociocultural sciences, in Comprehensive Textbook of Psychiatry, 6th Edition. Edited by Kaplan HI, Sadock BJ. Baltimore, MD, Williams & Wilkins, 1995, pp 337–354

C H A P T E R   4

Economic Issues in Child and Adolescent Psychiatry

Select the single best response for each question.

4.1   Which of the following is a strategy used by managed care organizations (MCOs) to contain costs for mental health services?

    A. Placing gatekeepers between patients and mental health providers.

    B. Requiring precertification.

    C. Channeling patients to the least expensive providers.

    D. Using prospective payment plans.

    E. All of the above.

The correct response is option E.

All of these cost-containment strategies have been used by MCOs to reduce access to and utilization of services by placing gatekeepers between patients and specialty services to limit referrals. Strategies include limiting utilization by requiring precertification or concurrent review of care and channeling patients from psychiatrists to less expensive mental health providers (e.g., social workers or psychologists). MCOs have also reversed the financial incentives inherent in retrospective fee-for-service reimbursement plans by using prospective payment plans, which require physicians and institutions to absorb the financial risk for the services they provide. A report by the Hay Group (1999) concluded that psychiatry has been more profoundly affected by these MCO strategies than has any other medical specialty. **(p. 59)**

4.2   Which of the following is an anticipated outcome of a single-payer health care financing model?

    A. Risk would be spread over a smaller segment of the population.

    B. Administrative overhead would most certainly increase.

    C. Payment for health care would shift from premium dollars to tax dollars.

    D. Uninsured people would be excluded from care.

    E. None of the above.

The correct response is option C.

Under single-payer financing, payment for health care would shift from premium dollars to tax dollars. The intent of single-payer financing is to spread risk over a larger, not smaller, segment of the population, to expand coverage to include many of the uninsured, and to reduce administrative overhead. **(p. 63)**

4.3   In the defined-contribution health plan arrangement, the employer

    A. Selects one health insurance plan for all employees.
    B. Carries over payments not used by employees to the next year.
    C. Provides a tax-sheltered account that may not be carried over to the next year.
    D. Caps the contribution it is willing to make.
    E. Remains the payer.

The correct response is option D.

The employer defines or caps the contribution it is willing to make toward the cost of the employee's health benefit. The employee, not the employer, selects a mix of health insurance options and other benefits to meet his or her needs. Employer contributions are made at the beginning of each year on a "use it or lose it" basis, and are not carried over into the next year. Under this arrangement, the employer ceases to be the payer and transfers the risks and responsibilities to the employee. **(p. 63)**

4.4   Disease management systems aim to promote wellness by managing risk in patients and in the population so as to improve outcomes in quality and cost of health care. Strategies employed to meet these goals include all of the following *except*

    A. Early detection of vulnerable individuals.
    B. Reliance on individual physician practice decisions.
    C. Patient education to empower self-management.
    D. Process and outcomes measurement, evaluation, and management.
    E. Use of a routine reporting/feedback loop.

The correct response is option B.

Rather than relying on decisions made by individual clinicians, disease management systems emphasize the use of evidence-based practice guidelines to manage risk in patients and to improve outcomes. Other goals are early detection of vulnerable individuals; close collaboration with physicians and support services; patient education; process and outcomes measurement, evaluation, and management; and use of a routine reporting/feedback loop. **(p. 64)**

4.5   According to Epidemiologic Catchment Area (ECA) study estimations, what percentage of Americans (including children and adolescents) in any given year had a diagnosable psychiatric disorder that required treatment?

    A. 5%.
    B. 10%.
    C. 15%.
    D. 20%.
    E. 25%.

The correct response is option D.

The ECA study revealed that in any given year, 20% of Americans, including children and adolescents, had a diagnosable psychiatric disorder that required treatment (Regier et al. 1993). It was further estimated that only 20% of the individuals who met diagnostic criteria received care. **(p. 66)**

References

Hay Group: Health care plan design and cost trends: 1988 through 1998. Report prepared for the National Association of Health Systems and the Association of Behavioral Group Practices. Arlington, VA, Hay Group, 1999

Regier DA, Narrow WE, Rae DS, et al: The de facto US mental and addictive disorders service system: Epidemiologic Catchment Area prospective 1-year prevalence rates of disorders and services. Arch Gen Psychiatry 50:85–94, 1993

CHAPTER 5

Classification of Child and Adolescent Psychiatric Disorders

Select the single best response for each question.

5.1   A number of changes were made in DSM-IV (American Psychiatric Association 1994) that apply to childhood. Which of the following is one of these changes?

   A. A new category of pervasive developmental disorders was to be coded on Axis II.
   B. Motor skills disorders were moved from Axis II to Axis I.
   C. Learning disorders were moved from Axis I to Axis II.
   D. Communications disorders were moved from Axis I to Axis II.
   E. None of the above.

The correct response is option B.

In DSM-IV, pervasive developmental disorders and learning disorders, motor skills disorder, and communication disorders were moved from Axis II to Axis I. **(p. 73)**

5.2   Pervasive developmental disorders include all of the following *except*

   A. Childhood schizophrenia.
   B. Autistic disorder.
   C. Rett's disorder.
   D. Asperger's disorder.
   E. Childhood disintegrative disorder.

The correct response is option A.

Childhood schizophrenia is not a pervasive developmental disorder. **(p. 73)**

5.3   In DSM-IV, the new category *feeding and eating disorders of infancy or early childhood* included all of the following *except*

   A. Feeding disorder of infancy or early childhood (persistent failure to eat adequately, with weight loss or failure to gain weight).
   B. Pica.
   C. Anorexia nervosa.
   D. Rumination disorder.
   E. None of the above.

The correct response is option C.

The new DSM-IV category *feeding and eating disorders of infancy or early childhood* included pica, rumination disorder, and feeding disorder of infancy or early childhood—the persistent failure to eat adequately and to gain weight. Anorexia nervosa and bulimia nervosa were moved to a separate eating disorders section. **(p. 74)**

5.4   The tic disorders category of DSM-IV was left essentially unchanged from that in DSM-III-R (American Psychiatric Association 1987) except for which of the following?

A. The addition of Tourette's disorder.
B. The elimination of chronic motor or vocal tic disorder.
C. The lowering of the upper limit of age at onset to 18 years.
D. The addition of transient tic disorder.
E. None of the above.

The correct response is option C.

The tic disorders category remained essentially unchanged in DSM-IV, with only a drop in the upper limit of age at onset from 21 to 18 years. The category includes Tourette's disorder, chronic motor or vocal tic disorder, transient tic disorder, and tic disorder not otherwise specified. **(p. 74)**

5.5   In DSM-IV, the category *other disorders of infancy, childhood, or adolescence* was reorganized to include which of the following disorders?

A. Separation anxiety disorder.
B. Selective mutism.
C. Reactive attachment disorder of infancy or early childhood.
D. Stereotypic movement disorder.
E. All of the above.

The correct response is option E.

In addition to all of the disorders listed above, the category *other disorders of infancy, childhood, or adolescence* contains a *not otherwise specified* diagnosis. **(p. 74)**

References

American Psychiatric Association: Diagnostic and Statistical Manual of Mental Disorders, 3rd Edition, Revised. Washington, DC, American Psychiatric Association, 1987

American Psychiatric Association: Diagnostic and Statistical Manual of Mental Disorders, 4th Edition. Washington, DC, American Psychiatric Association, 1994

C H A P T E R   6

Concepts of
Diagnostic Classification

Select the single best response for each question.

6.1   Knowledge of the diagnosis should allow the professional to make inferences about which of the
        following?

    A. Likely etiology of the disorder.
    B. Probable natural history of the disorder.
    C. Expected response of the disorder to specified types of treatment.
    D. The nature of other clinical conditions that are commonly associated with the disorder.
    E. All of the above.

The correct response is option E.

Knowledge of the diagnosis should allow the professional to make inferences about a disorder's likely
etiology, probable natural history, and expected response to specified types of treatment, as well as
about the nature of other clinical conditions that are commonly associated with the disorder. **(p. 79)**

6.2   Comorbidity between different diagnoses can arise for several reasons. Which of the following
        statements concerning potential causes of diagnostic comorbidity is *incorrect*?

    A. Comorbidity can arise as a result of purely structural factors, such as the presence of similar
        criteria in different disorders.
    B. Comorbidity can arise when two disorders lack an etiological relationship.
    C. Comorbidity can arise because the presence of one disorder has led to another as a complication.
    D. Comorbidity can arise because two disorders have common environmental or biological
        antecedents.
    E. All of the above.

The correct response is option B.

It is the presence—not absence—of an etiological relationship between two disorders that leads to
diagnostic comorbidity (e.g., the high rates of comorbidity between attention-deficit/hyperactivity
disorder [ADHD] and oppositional defiant disorder [ODD] may be attributable to the fact that
ADHD predisposes to ODD). In addition to the reasons listed in options A, C, and D above, a final
explanation for apparent comorbidity (of greatest concern for nosologists) is that it reflects errors of
diagnostic definition—that is, that the lines around different disorders have been drawn at the wrong
places and that what appear to be two commonly co-occurring disorders are, in reality, manifestations
of a single disorder. **(p. 80)**

6.3 DSM-IV-TR (American Psychiatric Association 2000) is an example of a categorical diagnostic system, in which a disorder is deemed either present or absent on the basis of whether an individual meets or does not meet certain criteria. Which of the following is an advantage of categorical diagnoses?

A. Disorders do not always present themselves in as complete a form as are represented by the diagnostic definitions.
B. Diagnostic criteria differ in their potential for causing impairment.
C. The number and type of symptoms will commonly vary with the age and sex of the patient.
D. The categorization of a disorder as being either present or absent represents the way that clinicians and patients think of disorders.
E. All of the above.

The correct response is option D.

An advantage of categorical systems is that they reflect the way that both clinicians and patients perceive disorders—that is, as being either present or absent. Although such a dichotomy is clear and seems precise, categorical diagnoses also involve certain distinct disadvantages, as stated in options A, B, and C above. **(p. 81)**

6.4 Which of the following is a disadvantage of dimensional/empirical diagnostic systems?

A. The items in the inventories are usually written in a complicated fashion with many qualifiers.
B. Factor structure remains constant across different age and gender groups.
C. Being a "case" becomes a function of deviation from normal scores rather than of impairment that interferes with functioning.
D. The information is usually collected from multiple instruments.
E. All of the above.

The correct response is option C.

In dimensional/empirical diagnostic systems, caseness (whether or not a disorder is deemed to be present) becomes a function of deviation from normal scores rather than a result of the degree of impairment or interference with functioning. Other disadvantages of dimensional/empirical diagnostic systems are that the items in the inventories are usually written simply, with few qualifiers; factor structure differs across different age and gender groups; and the information is usually collected with a single instrument, which means that scores on the individual factors or dimensions are usually highly correlated. **(p. 82)**

6.5 Because psychosocial circumstances and stressors may affect the diagnosis, treatment, and prognosis of psychiatric disorders, documenting the presence, history, and severity of such problems is important. It may, however, be difficult for patients to accurately recall the order of stressors and behavioral or emotional problems, because

A. Most childhood disorders are chronic.
B. The influence of subclinical premorbid states on an individual's functioning is difficult to reconstruct.
C. Many childhood stressors are chronic.
D. Distortions occur as part of a search for meaning.
E. All of the above.

The correct response is option E.

All of the reasons listed above are correct. **(p. 83)**

Reference

American Psychiatric Association: Diagnostic and Statistical Manual of Mental Disorders, 4th Edition, Text Revision. Washington, DC, American Psychiatric Association, 2000

C H A P T E R 7

Clinical Assessment in Infancy and Early Childhood

Select the single best response for each question.

7.1 Psychiatric clinical assessment in infancy

    A. Requires a less comprehensive approach than does assessment during childhood.
    B. Should focus most extensively on cognitive development.
    C. Requires evaluation of multiple lines of development.
    D. May exclude evaluation of risk factors.
    E. Is usually best conducted after the infant reaches 6 months of age.

The correct response is option C.

Psychiatric clinical assessment in infancy requires consideration of multiple lines of development—physical, cognitive, socioemotional, and familial. The psychiatric clinical assessment of an infant needs to be comprehensive; should include an evaluation of risk factors; and, ideally, should be conducted when a disturbance is first suspected, regardless of age. **(p. 87)**

7.2 Which of the following prenatal and perinatal variables should be assessed in infancy?

    A. Rubella.
    B. Maternal drug or alcohol use.
    C. Complications during pregnancy or delivery.
    D. Poor maternal nutrition.
    E. All of the above.

The correct response is option E.

All of the above prenatal and perinatal variables can affect an infant's constitutional status and development and thus should be assessed in infancy. **(p. 88)**

7.3 The stage-specific task of *representational capacity, differentiation, and consolidation* (the use of ideas to guide language, pretend play, and behavior) is mastered at which of the following ages?

    A. 0–3 months.
    B. 2–7 months.
    C. 3–10 months.
    D. 9–24 months.
    E. 1.5–4 years.

The correct response is option E.

Representation capacity, differentiation, and consolidation are mastered between the ages of 1.5 and 4 years. **(p. 91, Table 7–1)**

7.4   The developmental, individual-difference, relationship-based (DIR) model facilitates the process of clinical assessment in infancy and early childhood by identifying, systematizing, and integrating children's essential developmental capacities. These essential capacities include all of the following *except*

   A. The child's functional–emotional developmental level.
   B. The child's academic potential.
   C. The child's individual differences in sensory–affective processing.
   D. The child's relationships and interactions with caregivers and others.
   E. The child's individual differences in motor planning and sequencing.

The correct response is option B.

Essential functional developmental capacities of children include the capacities listed in options A, C, D, and E. Academic potential is not a part of the DIR model's core list of capacities. **(pp. 92–93)**

7.5   By the age of 12 months, a child would demonstrate all of the following capacities *except*

   A. Plays on own in a focused, organized manner for 15–20 minutes.
   B. Points and vocalizes at desired toy or object.
   C. Feeds self small finger foods.
   D. Throws a ball forward.
   E. Understands simple words or commands.

The correct response is option A.

By age 12 months, a child can usually play on his or her own, but only for about 10 minutes. By 18 months, the child can play independently for about 15 minutes; and by 2–2.5 years, for about 20 minutes. **(pp. 96–98, Table 7–2)**

C H A P T E R 8

The Clinical Interview
of the Child

Select the single best response for each question.

8.1 The Mental Health Assessment Form (MHAF)

   A. May be used with children between the ages of 3 and 6 years.
   B. Usually requires about 3 hours to complete.
   C. Employs questionnaires.
   D. Consists of 54 items.
   E. Obtains information on all areas of a child's life and functioning.

   The correct response is option E.

   The MHAF (Kestenbaum and Bird 1978) was developed to provide a bridge between the structured questionnaire and the open-ended clinical interview. It consists of 189 items, can be used with children between the ages of 6 and 12 years, does not employ questionnaires or cards, and is designed to gather information on all areas of the child's life and functioning. **(pp. 104–105)**

8.2 The MHAF consists of two parts. Part II ("Content of the Interview") deals with all of the following areas *except*

   A. Motoric behavior and speech.
   B. Interpersonal relations.
   C. Self-concept.
   D. Feeling states.
   E. Symbolic representation.

   The correct response is option A.

   Motoric behavior and speech are addressed in Part I ("Mental Status"), not Part II, of the MHAF. In addition to the areas listed above, Part II also deals with conscience/moral judgment and the child's general level of adaptation. **(p. 105)**

8.3 When interviewing the younger child (ages 5–9 years), the examiner should do all of the following *except*

   A. Interview one or both parents before meeting the child.
   B. Allow the child to examine the environment.
   C. Explain the nature of the interview to the parents.
   D. Refrain from explaining the reason for the interview to the child, because such information may be upsetting.
   E. Provide reassurance if necessary.

The correct response is option D.

The clinician should interview one or both parents before meeting the child, in order to ascertain the nature of the presenting problem and to obtain pertinent information; should allow the child to examine the surroundings; and should explain to the child the reason for the interview, providing reassurance if necessary. **(p. 106)**

8.4   When interviewing the older child (ages 10–12 years), the examiner should

    A. Begin with general questions to avoid having a child get defensive about the chief complaint.
    B. Start by using the MHAF designed for older children.
    C. Obtain some idea about the child's development of empathy.
    D. End with the chief complaint.
    E. Refrain from having a parents-only meeting after the initial interview so that the child will not feel excluded.

The correct response is option C.

The interviewer should begin with the chief complaint and should attempt to assess the extent of the child's development of empathy by asking questions about family pets and other animals. There is no specific age cutoff at which the "older children" version of MHAF should be used; the decision depends on the child's cognitive level as assessed by the interviewer. The treatment plan may or may not include separate parents-only or child-only meetings. However, older children should be told of the expected plan either way. **(pp. 109–110)**

8.5   The MHAF semistructured interview can be used to accomplish all of the following *except*

    A. Assess for the signs and symptoms of a psychiatric disorder.
    B. Identify positive attributes of the patient.
    C. Conduct a formal assessment of the patient's cognitive functioning.
    D. Establish a relationship with the patient.
    E. Evaluate the strengths of the patient.

The correct response is option C.

The MHAF is not designed to obtain a formal assessment of cognitive functioning. **(p. 110)**

Reference

Kestenbaum CJ, Bird HR: A reliability study of the Mental Health Assessment Form for school-age children. J Am Acad Child Psychiatry 17:338–347, 1978

C H A P T E R   9

The Clinical Interview
of the Adolescent

Select the single best response for each question.

9.1   Which of the following statements concerning the initial interview of an adolescent is *false?*

A. Seeing the adolescent first highlights the patient's active participation in the process.
B. Seeing the adolescent first may allay fears that the parents and therapist will gang up on the patient.
C. The therapeutic alliance between the clinician and adolescent may be harmed if the clinician meets alone with the parents; such an approach is therefore discouraged.
D. The clinician should make clear to the adolescent that he or she is not out to assign blame.
E. None of the above.

The correct response is option C.

Several factors must be considered when deciding whether the initial meeting should be with the adolescent, the parents, or all together. In most cases, the adolescent should be present at the first meeting, preferably alone, in order to encourage his or her active participation. However, it is also important to meet with the parents alone at some point so that the clinician can obtain information that would be difficult to obtain with the adolescent present. **(p. 113)**

9.2   Characteristic adolescent patterns of responding to interviews with a therapist include which of the following?

A. Anxiety about revealing problems that they may regard as weaknesses.
B. Externalization of one side or another of conflicted feelings.
C. Counterphobic measures to deal with painful affects.
D. An unrealistic faith in the "omnipotence of thought."
E. All of the above.

The correct response is option E.

In addition to all of the above considerations, it is good to remember that the adolescent's relationship with most adults is colored by a strong push toward autonomy and a great wariness of feeling vulnerable, dependent, or controlled. **(p. 114)**

9.3   To interview an adolescent effectively, which of the following are important qualities for a clinician?

A. Having experienced similar problems in adolescence.
B. Possessing a sense of humor.
C. Being informal and familiar.
D. Being close in age to the adolescent so that he or she can identify with the clinician.
E. All of the above.

The correct response is option B.

Of the qualities listed, only a sense of humor is important. Having experienced similar struggles is not helpful unless the clinician has actually come to terms with the problems of his or her own adolescence. A skilled clinician can be effective regardless of his or her age. **(pp. 114–115)**

9.4   When should a formal mental status examination be conducted with an adolescent?

A. When there is a concern about psychosis.
B. When the disorder may be severe.
C. When precise documentation is required.
D. When there is a possibility of dementia.
E. All of the above.

The correct response is option E.

A formal mental status exam should be conducted when the disorder is severe, when precise documentation is required, or when there are concerns about psychosis, dementia, or an organic brain syndrome. **(p. 115)**

9.5   In interviewing adolescents, the therapist should

A. Limit the interview to areas of difficulty.
B. Demonstrate his or her familiarity with any topic that the adolescent may bring up, such as rock groups.
C. Make early interpretations to assist the adolescent with the session.
D. Avoid asking about dating or sexual relationships.
E. Ask about friends and peers.

The correct response is option E.

An important area of exploration with adolescents is that of friends and peers, which will lead naturally to the topic of dating and sexual relationships. The interview should not be limited to areas of difficulty. It is better to simply let the adolescent express his or her particular interests, rather than attempting to demonstrate one's own familiarity with the topics. In addition, the clinician should resist the temptation to make early interpretations—such communications are more likely to scare the patient away than to be helpful. **(pp. 115–116)**

C H A P T E R 1 0

The Parent Interview

Select the single best response for each question.

10.1   Mednick and Shaffer (1963) found that when maternal interviews were compared with pediatric records, the mothers' reports were discrepant what percentage of the time?

A. 0–6%.
B. 7%–15%.
C. 16%–20%.
D. 21%–62%.
E. 63%–75%.

The correct response is option D.

When maternal interviews were compared with pediatric records, the mothers' reports were found to be discrepant 21%–62% of the time for facts about discrete experiences, such as breast-feeding, childhood illnesses, and the age at completion of toilet training (Mednick and Shaffer 1963). **(pp. 117–118)**

10.2   A number of investigators have studied the parent interview. Which of the following descriptions of their findings is *incorrect*?

A. Weissman et al. (1987) found that parents reported far more information about their children's disorders than did the children themselves.
B. Orvaschel et al. (1981) found that parents were more accurate in providing factual time-related information.
C. Edelbrock et al. (1985) found that the reliability of a child's report increased with the child's age.
D. Edelbrock et al. (1985) found that in children 10 years of age and older, parent and child reports showed little or no difference in reliability.
E. None of the above.

The correct response is option A.

Weissman at al. (1987) found that children reported far more information about their disorders than did their parents. **(p. 118)**

10.3   Which of the following is a function of the parent interview?

A. Gathering information about the child's history.
B. Assessing the child's present functioning.
C. Identifying the child's strengths and weaknesses.
D. Giving parents information about normal child development.
E. All of the above.

The correct response is option E.

All of the above are important functions of the parent interview. **(p. 118)**

10.4   The parent interview may be divided into five phases: preliminaries, prologue, interview proper, closing, and epilogue. What is the primary purpose of the *closing* phase?

A. Assess the parents' and the clinician's expectations for the interview.
B. Establish an alliance or empathetic relationship with the parents while collecting data and making the appropriate interventions.
C. Reassure the parents and reinforce their control and competence.
D. Review the interview, the validity of the plans, and the next step.
E. None of the above.

The correct response is option C.

The purpose of the *closing* phase is to reassure the parents and reinforce their control and competence. The purpose of the *preliminaries* phase is to identify the patient and the purpose of the interview. During the *prologue*, it is useful to assess both the parents' and the clinician's expectations for the interview. The *interview proper* provides the opportunity to establish an alliance with the parents while collecting data and making the appropriate interventions. During the *epilogue*, the clinician can review the validity of the plans and the next step. **(pp. 119–120)**

10.5   In emergency settings, the focus of the parent interview is

A. Directly related to the parents' sense of control, frustration, and incompetence in the clinical situation.
B. To assess the risk of danger and to establish a safe and protective environment for the child.
C. To assess the child's medical care.
D. To obtain factual and impressionistic information.
E. All of the above.

The correct response is option B.

In emergency settings, the focus of the interview must be on assessing the risk of danger and establishing a safe and protective environment for the child. **(p. 121)**

References

Edelbrock C, Costello AJ, Dulcan NM, et al: Age differences in the reliability of the psychiatric interview of the child. Child Dev 56:265–275, 1985

Mednick SA, Shaffer JBP: Mothers' retrospective reports in child-rearing research. Am J Orthopsychiatry 33:457–461, 1963

Orvaschel H, Weissman MM, Padian N, et al: Assessing psychopathology in children of psychiatrically disturbed parents: a pilot study. J Am Acad Child Psychiatry 20:112–122, 1981

Weissman MM, Wickramaratne P, Warner V, et al: Assessing psychiatric disorders in children: discrepancies between mothers' and children's reports. Arch Gen Psychiatry 44:747–753, 1987

CHAPTER 11

Initial and Diagnostic Family Interviews

Select the single best response for each question.

11.1 The diagnostic family interview is commonly divided into three segments: 1) social stage, 2) multidimensional inquiry into the presenting problem, and 3) exploration of the structure and developmental phase of the family. During the *multidimensional inquiry stage* of the initial family interview

    A. The clinician initiates the engagement by serving as host to the family.
    B. The clinician does not yet address the presenting problem.
    C. The clinician should be prepared to encounter family resistance to broadening the focus of the discussion.
    D. The clinical assessment of the family's developmental level is of primary importance.
    E. The clinician focuses on the functional adequacy of various family subsystems.

The correct response is option C.

The clinician should be prepared to encounter resistance from the family members against broadening the focus of the explorations and discussing potentially uncomfortable details of the presenting problem. In the *multidimensional inquiry* stage, the clinician asks the family to describe the presenting problem. The clinician acts as a host to the family during the *social stage* of the interview, not the multidimensional inquiry stage. Assessment of the functional adequacy of family subsystems occurs during the stage of *exploration of family structure*. **(p. 126)**

11.2 Which of the following is *not* considered an accepted therapist function during family assessment?

    A. Understanding the roles of the different family members.
    B. Uncovering explicit and implicit family rules.
    C. Determining the family's typical problem-solving strategies.
    D. Understanding the nature of boundaries, splits, and alliances among family members.
    E. Allying with healthier family members during discussions with less healthy members.

The correct response is option E.

The therapist should not ally with healthier family members in discussions with less healthy members. **(p. 128)**

11.3   The family life-cycle stage of "becoming three" is best defined as

A. Establishment of a common household by two adults.
B. Development of parental identity.
C. Arrival and inclusion of the first child.
D. Exit of the oldest child from the family during late adolescence.
E. Death of a spouse.

The correct response is option C.

Stage II of the early stages of the family cycle, known as "becoming three," is initiated by the arrival and subsequent inclusion of the first child into the family. **(p. 131, Table 11–1)**

11.4   Which of the following is *not* one of Minuchin's (1974) major areas of family assessment?

A. The family structure.
B. The family financial status.
C. The family system's flexibility.
D. The family life context.
E. The family developmental stage.

The correct response is option B.

The family financial status is not one of the major areas of family assessment according to Minuchin (1974). **(p. 132)**

11.5   Which of the following family rating scales, widely used in research, measures the social climate of all types of families, with subscales in the areas of family cohesion, expressiveness, conflict, independence, and achievement?

A. The Family Environment Scale.
B. The Card Sorting Procedure.
C. The Family Adaptability Cohesion Evaluation Scale.
D. The Beavers-Timberlawn Family Evaluation Scale.
E. The Family Assessment Device.

The correct response is option A.

The Family Environment Scale (Moos and Moos 1980) measures social climates of all types of families, with various subscales. It has been used widely in many research projects. The other scales listed above assess additional aspects of family dynamics. **(p. 133)**

References

Minuchin S: Families and Family Therapy. Cambridge, MA, Harvard University Press, 1974

Moos R, Moos B: Family Environment Scale Manual. Palo Alto, CA, Consulting Psychologists Press, 1980

C H A P T E R   1 2

Diagnostic Interviews

Select the single best response for each question.

12.1   According to Angold and Fisher (1999), clinician diagnoses are potentially fraught with numerous biases. All of the following are examples of such biases *except*

   A. Making diagnoses before all relevant information is collected.
   B. Collecting information selectively when confirming and/or ruling out a diagnosis.
   C. Not systematically collecting and organizing information.
   D. Not permitting one's special expertise to influence diagnostic assessment.
   E. Assuming correlations in symptoms and illnesses that in reality are spurious or nonexistent.

The correct response is option D.

By allowing his or her own special expertise to influence diagnostic assessment, a clinician would potentially bias the diagnosis. **(p. 138)**

12.2   *Construct validity* is defined as

   A. How well a category as defined appears to describe a recognized illness.
   B. Whether a category has meaning in terms of what it is designed to describe.
   C. How well a category predicts a pertinent aspect of care.
   D. How internally consistent a measure is.
   E. How often different interviewers assign the same diagnosis.

The correct response is option B.

Construct validity refers to whether a category has meaning in terms of what it is designed to describe. *Face validity* is how well a category appears to describe an illness. *Predictive validity* is how well the category predicts a pertinent aspect of care. *Reliability* is how internally consistent the measure is, and *interrater reliability* is how often different interviewers assign the same diagnosis. **(p. 139)**

12.3   Which of the statements concerning reliability is *false?*

   A. Reliability includes how often different interviewers assign the same diagnosis.
   B. Diagnostic tools need to be reliable in order to be useful.
   C. Reliability ensures validity.
   D. Reliability includes how internally consistent the measure is.
   E. Reliability encompasses how consistently respondents report the same symptoms or diagnoses over time.

The correct response is option C.

Reliability does not ensure validity. A diagnostic category may be reliably defined but not valid. Conversely, a disorder may be valid, but the diagnostic criteria or the instruments used to assess for its presence may not be reliable. **(p. 139)**

12.4 Which of the following statements concerning assessment of a diagnostic instrument's ability to detect cases is *true?*

A. *Sensitivity* is the percentage of individuals in a sample who have the disorder who are accurately identified by the interview.

B. *Predictive value positive* is the percentage of individuals in the defined sample positively identified by the interview who actually have the disorder.

C. *Specificity* is the percentage of individuals in a sample who do not have the disorder who are accurately identified by the interview as not having the disorder.

D. *Predictive value negative* is the percentage of individuals in the defined sample identified as not having the disorder by the interview who in fact do not have the disorder.

E. All of the above.

The correct response is option E.

All of the above definitions are correct. **(p. 140)**

12.5 Although a number of structured diagnostic interviews are available for assessment of psychiatric illnesses in youth, these instruments have limitations. Examples of such limitations include all of the following *except*

A. Children may underreport new or unusual phenomena.

B. Children may lack the requisite attention span.

C. Children may lack the abstract awareness to understand the concepts.

D. Children may not be aware of the concept being described.

E. Children may lack the necessary verbal skills.

The correct response is option A.

Children tend to overreport, not underreport, rare or unusual phenomena, such as obsessive-compulsive, psychotic, or manic symptoms. **(p. 145)**

Reference

Angold A, Fisher PW: Interviewer-based interviews, in Diagnostic Assessment in Child and Adolescent Psychopathology. Edited by Shaffer D, Lucas CP, Richters JE. New York, Guilford, 1999, pp 34–64

C H A P T E R   1 3

Rating Scales

Select the single best response for each question.

13.1   The *reliability* of a rating instrument

   A. Is equivalent to random error.
   B. Refers to the consistency with which an instrument measures a construct in the same way every time.
   C. Pertains to whether the instrument accurately assesses what it was designed to measure.
   D. Is inversely proportional to the validity of the instrument.
   E. Is reduced when the measured construct changes over time.

   The correct response is option B.

   Reliability refers to the consistency with which a scale's items measure the same construct every time. **(p. 150)**

13.2   Which of the following is the best example of a broad-band rating scale?

   A. Conners Rating Scale—Revised.
   B. Children's Depression Inventory.
   C. Hopelessness Scale for Children.
   D. Child Behavior Checklist.
   E. ADHD Rating Scale–IV.

   The correct response is option D.

   The Child Behavior Checklist (Achenbach and Rescorla 2000, 2001) is the most popular broad-band rating scale and has been considered the "gold standard" since the 1960s. **(p. 150)**

13.3   All of the following statements pertaining to broad-band rating scales are correct *except*

   A. They include measurements of both internalizing and externalizing behaviors.
   B. They assess a variety of clinical problems.
   C. They may be lengthy and cumbersome to complete.
   D. They assess for both breadth and depth of pathology in all clinical domains.
   E. They are best used to identify problems that will require further evaluation.

   The correct response is option D.

   Broad-band scales tend to sacrifice depth of assessment for breadth. **(pp. 150–152)**

13.4 The Conners Rating Scale—Revised

   A. Includes parent, teacher, and youth self-report versions.
   B. Mostly assesses internalizing behaviors.
   C. Includes some abbreviated versions, but only for youth self-report.
   D. Has no mechanism for assessing common comorbid conditions.
   E. Is most useful for initial assessment in its abbreviated version.

   The correct response is option A.

   The Conners Rating Scale—Revised (Conners 1997), the primary attention-deficit/hyperactivity disorder (ADHD) rating scale, includes parent, teacher, and youth self-report versions. **(pp. 153–155, Table 13–2)**

13.5 Which of the following scales measuring internalizing symptoms is clinician-administered rather than self-reported?

   A. Beck Depression Inventory.
   B. Children's Depression Inventory.
   C. Children's Depression Rating Scale.
   D. Beck Hopelessness Scale.
   E. Hopelessness Scale for Children.

   The correct response is option C.

   The Children's Depression Rating Scale—Revised (Poznanski and Mokros 1999) is administered by a clinician, a feature thought to provide greater accuracy than is possible with self-report or adult-report instruments. **(p. 157, Table 13–3)**

References

Achenbach TM, Rescorla LA: Manual for the ASEBA school-age forms & profiles. Burlington, VT, University of Vermont, Research Center for Children, Youth, and Families, 2000. Available from the Achenbach System of Empirically Based Assessment (ASEBA), 1 South Prospect Street, room 6436, Burlington, VT 05401-3456; phone: (802) 656-8313 or (802) 656-2608; http://www.aseba.org. Accessed May 1, 2003.

Achenbach TM, Rescorla LA: Manual for the ASEBA preschool forms & profiles. Burlington, VT, University of Vermont, Research Center for Children, Youth, and Families, 2001. Available from the Achenbach System of Empirically Based Assessment (ASEBA), 1 South Prospect Street, room 6436, Burlington, VT 05401-3456; phone: (802) 656-8313 or (802) 656-2608; http://www.aseba.org. Accessed May 1, 2003.

Conners CK: Conners' Rating Scales—Revised, Technical Manual. North Tonawanda, NY, Multi-Health Systems, 1997. Available from Multi-Health Systems, Inc., 908 Niagara Falls Boulevard, North Tonawanda, NY 14120-2060; (800) 456-3003; http://www.mhs.com. Accessed April 30, 2003.

Poznanski EO, Mokros HB: Children's Depression Rating Scale—Revised (CDRS-R). Los Angeles, CA, Western Psychological Services, 1999. Available from Western Psychological Services, 12031 Wilshire Boulevard 90025-1251; phone: (800) 648-8857; http://www.wpspublish.com. Accessed May 2, 2003.

C H A P T E R   1 4

Psychological and Neuropsychological Testing

Select the single best response for each question.

14.1   Which of the following statements concerning intelligence tests is *true*?

    A. Intelligence test scores vary widely for children over the age of 5 years.
    B. IQ scores are strong predictors of overall adjustment.
    C. IQ scores are strongly associated with academic achievement.
    D. All of the above.
    E. None of the above.

The correct response is option C.

IQ scores are strongly associated with academic achievement but are only modestly predictive of overall adjustment. Scores from intelligence tests are quite stable for children older than 5 years.
(p. 169)

14.2   According to DSM-IV-TR (American Psychiatric Association 2000), an individual is identified as being mentally retarded if, in addition to being functionally impaired, he or she has a standardized IQ score below

    A. 90.
    B. 70.
    C. 50.
    D. 30.
    E. None of the above.

The correct response is option B.

Individuals are identified as being mentally retarded if their standardized IQ score is below 70.
(p. 170)

14.3   Which of the following instruments measures intellectual and cognitive functioning in children and adolescents?

    A. McCarthy Scales of Children's Abilities.
    B. Kaufman Assessment Battery for Children.
    C. Leiter International Performance Scale—Revised.
    D. Differential Abilities Scale.
    E. All of the above.

The correct response is option E.

All of the above instruments are measures of intellectual and cognitive functioning for children and adolescents. **(p. 171, Table 14–2)**

14.4　All of the following are measures of socioemotional functioning in children and adolescents *except*

A.　Gestalt Closure Test.
B.　Children's Apperception Test.
C.　Rorschach Inkblot Test.
D.　Sentence-completion test.
E.　Human Figure Drawing.

The correct response is option A.

The Gestalt Closure Test is a measure of *perceptual* function for children and adolescents, not a measure of socioemotional functioning. **(pp. 173, 175; Tables 14–4, 14–7)**

Reference

American Psychiatric Association: Diagnostic and Statistical Manual of Mental Disorders, 4th Edition, Text Revision. Washington, DC, American Psychiatric Association, 2000

CHAPTER 15

Laboratory and Diagnostic Testing

Select the single best response for each question.

15.1   In a study conducted by Sheline and Kehr (1990), the use of screening tests in psychiatric inpatients led to changes in clinical management in what percentage of cases?

A. 1%.
B. 6%.
C. 10%.
D. 14%.
E. None of the above.

The correct response is option B.

Although 49% of the patients had coexisting medical illnesses, laboratory tests led to changes in clinical management for only 6% of these patients (Sheline and Kehr 1990). **(p. 183)**

15.2   Laboratory tests recommended as part of a comprehensive examination or premedication workup include all of the following *except*

A. Complete blood count (CBC).
B. Urinalysis.
C. Thyroid panel.
D. Liver function tests.
E. Blood urea nitrogen (BUN).

The correct response is option C.

A thyroid panel is not part of the recommended workup. The following tests are recommended: CBC, differential and hematocrit; urinalysis; BUN level; serum electrolytes; liver function tests; and lead level in children younger than 7 years of age when risk factors are present or in older children when indicated. **(p. 183)**

15.3   Which of the following thyroid disorders has been reported to be associated with attention-deficit/hyperactivity disorder (ADHD)–like symptoms?

A. Hyperthyroidism.
B. Syndrome of resistance to thyroid hormone.
C. Hypothyroidism.
D. All of the above.
E. None of the above.

The correct response is option D.

All three thyroid disorders listed above have been reported to be associated with ADHD-like symptoms. **(p. 185)**

15.4 For patients who attempt suicide by drug overdose, recommended medical/laboratory tests depend on the specific substance taken. Which of the following recommendations is *incorrect?*

    A. Blood toxicology workup for overdose on illegal substances.
    B. Liver function test for acetaminophen overdose.
    C. Serum electrolytes for aspirin overdose.
    D. Electrocardiogram (ECG) for selective serotonin reuptake inhibitor (SSRI) overdose.
    E. None of the above.

The correct response is option D.

An ECG should be obtained for patients who have overdosed with tricyclic antidepressants (TCAs), not necessarily SSRIs, unless the patient has a history of underlying cardiac problems. Blood toxicology workups should be ordered for patients who have overdosed on prescribed drugs or illegal substances. Liver function tests are important for assessing acetaminophen overdose, and serum electrolyte values are needed to assess anion gap in cases of aspirin overdose. **(p. 185)**

15.5 Peer-reviewed articles support the use of single-photon emission computed tomography (SPECT) to rule out which of the following disorders in children?

    A. ADHD.
    B. Wilson's disease.
    C. Seizure disorder.
    D. Prader-Willi syndrome.
    E. None of the above.

The correct response is option E.

The peer-reviewed scientific literature contains no analyses of the validity of SPECT in the diagnosis and treatment of neurodevelopmental disorders. **(p. 187)**

Reference

Sheline Y, Kehr C: Cost and utility of routine admission laboratory testing for psychiatric inpatients. Gen Hosp Psychiatry 12:329–334, 1990

C H A P T E R   1 6

Clinical Genomic Testing

Select the single best response for each question.

16.1   Which of the following statements concerning the cytochrome P450 *2D6* gene is *false?*

A. It is primarily responsible for the metabolism of many psychotropic medications such as fluoxetine, paroxetine, and selected tricyclic antidepressants.
B. It is located on the long arm of chromosome 22.
C. Unlike other cytochrome P450 genes, it has few polymorphisms.
D. It metabolizes codeine.
E. None of the above.

The correct response is option C.

The cytochrome P450 *2D6* gene is one of the most highly variable genes. More than 70 variants have been reported. **(p. 194)**

16.2   Polymorphisms associated with which of the following dopamine transporter or receptor genes have been found in selected families with a well-documented history of schizophrenia?

A. Dopamine transporter gene.
B. Dopamine receptor 2 gene.
C. Dopamine receptor 3 gene.
D. Dopamine receptor 4 gene.
E. None of the above.

The correct response is option C.

The dopamine 3 receptor (*DRD3*) gene, located on the long arm of the third chromosome, has been linked to schizophrenia. **(pp. 195–196)**

16.3   Polymorphisms of the serotonin transporter (*5HTT*) gene have been reported to be associated with all of the following *except*

A. Obsessive-compulsive disorder.
B. Suicidal behavior in depressed patients.
C. Autism.
D. Attention-deficit/hyperactivity disorder (ADHD).
E. Increased fear- and anxiety-related symptoms.

The correct response is option D.

The *5HTT* gene has been linked to obsessive-compulsive disorder, to suicide in depressed patients, to autism, and to increased fear- and anxiety-related behaviors, but not to ADHD. **(pp. 196–197)**

16.4 Polymorphisms of the tryptophan hydroxylase (*TPH*) gene have been linked to all of the following *except*

A. Suicidal behavior.
B. Bipolar disorder.
C. Early smoking initiation.
D. Panic disorder.
E. Alcohol abuse.

The correct response is option D.

Polymorphisms of the *TPH* gene have not been linked to panic disorder. **(pp. 197–198)**

16.5 Critical elements of medical testing that also apply to genomic testing include all of the following *except*

A. There should be adequate informed consent.
B. Testing need not be voluntary.
C. Test results must be accurate.
D. Information obtained from the test must provide some potential medical or psychological benefit.
E. The patient should be provided with information on both benefits and risks.

The correct response is option B.

The decision to have a test must be voluntary. Other principles guiding both genomic and medical testing are that there must be adequate informed consent, with information regarding both benefits and risks provided to the patient; test results must be accurate; and knowledge derived from the test must provide some potential medical or psychological benefit. **(p. 199)**

C H A P T E R   1 7

Diagnosis and Diagnostic Formulation

Select the single best response for each question.

17.1   The psychiatric formulation of a child's case

A. Must simultaneously consider biological, social, developmental, and psychological contributing factors.
B. Requires access to one or two sources of information.
C. Is a relatively simple process.
D. May not require consideration of social factors in some cases.
E. Requires that the child be viewed as separate and distinct from his or her family network.

The correct response is option A.

The psychiatric formulation of a child's case must simultaneously consider biological, social, developmental, and psychological factors. Appropriate case formulation is complex, requires multiple sources of information, and necessitates a consideration of social factors. **(p. 205)**

17.2   Which of the following statements regarding the Diagnostic and Statistical Manual (DSM) is *true?*

A. The DSM clarifies the etiology for most disorders.
B. The DSM incorporates multiple theoretical paradigms in defining disorder caseness.
C. The use of DSM typically results in low comorbidity of psychiatric diagnoses in the child population.
D. The DSM requires descriptive symptomatology to qualify for diagnosis using established criteria.
E. Resultant DSM diagnoses link to precise and effective treatments.

The correct response is option D.

The DSM follows a diagnostic approach that is based on cross-sectional categories which describe specific syndromes on Axis I. The DSM offers little guidance about etiology and nosology of disorders. Dimensional issues, for instance, which are so vital to a developmental point of view of childhood, are excluded. When a child receives a psychiatric diagnosis, it is important to note the developmental status of the child so as to account for the effect of immaturity in coping mechanisms on the diagnosis and the rapidity of behavioral regression and recovery. Both children and adults have high rates of psychiatric comorbidity. **(p. 206)**

17.3   Which of the following statements concerning DSM-IV-TR (2000) developmental disorders is *false?*

A. The category includes pervasive developmental disorders and autism.
B. The category does not include mental retardation.
C. Diagnoses in this category are coded on Axis II.

D. Typically, disorders in this category are characterized by an uneven or deviant developmental profile.
E. These disorders commonly co-occur with other conditions.

The correct response is option C.

The developmental disorders category is coded on Axis I, not Axis II, and includes pervasive developmental disorders, autism, learning disabilities, and attention-deficit/hyperactivity disorder (ADHD). Mental retardation is coded on Axis II. Disorders in this category show a deviant or uneven developmental pattern. Comorbidity is prominent in childhood. **(pp. 208–209)**

17.4 In cataloging the relevant biological features of a child's case, important factors to consider include all of the following *except*

A. Family genetic history.
B. Early caregiving practices.
C. Language disorder history in first-degree relatives.
D. Early childhood meningitis.
E. Malnutrition.

The correct response is option B.

Early caregiving practices are important *environmental*, not biological, features of a child's case. Important *biological* features for clinicians to consider are other familial factors (including diseases and disorders in first-degree relatives, genetic history, and developmental delays within the family) and early childhood infections or toxic-metabolic states such as meningitis, viral encephalitis, diabetic coma, or malnutrition. **(p. 210)**

17.5 Which of the following statements concerning psychodynamic formulations is *false?*

A. The presence of unconscious functioning is assumed.
B. Unconscious internal conflicts typically contribute to symptom formation.
C. Symptoms have psychological meaning to the child.
D. Presenting problems are driven to expression within the transference relationship with the therapist.
E. Nondynamic factors are extraneous to the formulation.

The correct response is option E.

Nondynamic factors are intrinsic to psychodynamic formulation. Four fundamental notions are essential to dynamic formulation: the presence of unconscious functioning is assumed; unconscious internal conflicts typically contribute to symptom formation; symptoms have psychological meaning to the child; and a central need exists to displace internalized conflicts and maladaptive interpersonal relationships onto the therapist as transferential behaviors. **(p. 211)**

Reference

American Psychiatric Association: Diagnostic and Statistical Manual of Mental Disorders, 4th Edition, Text Revision. Washington, DC, American Psychiatric Association, 2000

C H A P T E R   1 8

Presentation of Findings and Recommendations

Select the single best response for each question.

18.1   The main purposes of the postassessment or "informing" interview in regard to a child or adolescent patient include which of the following?

A. Sharing the clinician's observation with the child's parents.
B. Elaborating further on parental feelings and perceptions.
C. Discussing the clinician's recommendations.
D. Arriving at a plan that will be helpful to the child and the family.
E. All of the above.

The correct response is option E.

The postassessment interview is a crucial aspect of the diagnostic process in child and adolescent psychiatry. Its main purposes are to share the clinician's observation with the child's parents, to elaborate further on parental feelings and perceptions, and to discuss the clinician's recommendations so as to arrive collaboratively at a treatment plan. **(p. 215)**

18.2   Which of the following statements concerning confidentiality in children and adolescents is *false?*

A. Confidentiality is qualitatively different for younger children than for adolescents.
B. The clinician can promise confidentiality to a child with the proviso that information that is potentially self-destructive or destructive to others will be shared with those who may protect the child.
C. It is usually necessary to include younger children in the postdiagnostic interview.
D. The issues of confidentiality are of greater importance to adolescent patients than they are for adult patients.
E. None of the above.

The correct response is option C.

It usually is not necessary to include younger children in the postdiagnostic interview. **(p. 217)**

18.3   Factors that are relevant to a family's remaining in therapy include all of the following *except*

A. The therapist's activity and directiveness.
B. The family's ability to influence the consultation.
C. The congruence between the family's expectations and the therapist's response.
D. The severity of the child's psychiatric disorder.
E. The family's perception that they are active participants in the therapeutic process.

The correct response is option D.

The family's relationship with the therapist and the therapist's directedness, not the severity of the child's disorder, usually determine whether the family remains in therapy. **(p. 218)**

C H A P T E R   1 9

Mental Retardation

Select the single best response for each question.

19.1   DSM-IV-TR (American Psychiatric Association 2000) criteria require an IQ score in which of the following ranges for a diagnosis of "severe mental retardation"?

A. Below 20–25.
B. Between 20–25 and 35–40.
C. Between 35–40 and 50–55.
D. Between 50–55 and 70.
E. None of the above.

The correct response is option B.

The diagnosis of severe mental retardation requires an IQ score between 20–25 and 35–40. **(p. 224, Table 19–1)**

19.2   Data from the National Health Interview Survey for 1994–1995 (University of Minnesota 2000) indicate that the combined prevalence of mental retardation and developmental disabilities in the United States during that period was approximately what percentage of the population?

A. 1.5%.
B. 3%.
C. 5%.
D. 7%.
E. 9%.

The correct response is option A.

The prevalence of mental retardation and developmental disabilities in the United States in 1994–1995 was 1.58% (University of Minnesota 2000). **(p. 224)**

19.3   Prader-Willi syndrome in children is characterized by all of the following *except*

A. Obesity.
B. Hypogonadism in males.
C. Spasticity.
D. Dysmorphic features.
E. Hyperphagia.

The correct response is option C.

Prader-Willi syndrome is not characterized by spasticity, but rather by hypotonia, obesity, developmental and behavioral problems (including mental retardation), hyperphagia, hypogonadism in males, and dysmorphic features. **(p. 234, Table 19–4)**

19.4 DNA probes and molecular biology analyses have identified the q11–q12 region of chromosome 15 as the abnormal region of the human genome responsible for which of the following syndromes?

    A. Prader-Willi syndrome and Angelman's syndrome.
    B. Angelman's syndrome and fragile X syndrome.
    C. Prader-Willi syndrome and fragile X syndrome.
    D. Prader-Willi syndrome and Williams syndrome.
    E. Fragile X syndrome and Rett's disorder.

The correct response is option A.

Abnormalities of the q11–q12 region of chromosome 15 have been implicated in Prader-Willi and Angelman's syndromes. **(p. 234)**

19.5 The most common inherited form of mental retardation is

    A. Angelman's syndrome.
    B. Rett's disorder.
    C. Williams syndrome.
    D. Prader-Willi syndrome.
    E. Fragile X syndrome.

The correct response is option E.

Fragile X syndrome is the most common inherited form of mental retardation. **(p. 235)**

19.6 Current estimates of the prevalence of schizophrenia in individuals with mental retardation are in the range of

    A. 1%–3%.
    B. 3%–5%.
    C. 5%–8%.
    D. 8%–10%.
    E. 10%–12%.

The correct response is option A.

Current estimates of the prevalence of schizophrenia in persons with mental retardation range from 1% to 2%–3%. **(pp. 247–248)**

References

American Psychiatric Association: Diagnostic and Statistical Manual of Mental Disorders, 4th Edition, Text Revision. Washington, DC, American Psychiatric Association, 2000

University of Minnesota, the College of Education and Human Development: MR/DD Data Brief, Vol 2, No. 1, p 5, 2000. Available at: http://rtc.umn.edu/nhis/databrief2/index.html. Accessed July 2003.

C H A P T E R   2 0

Autistic Disorder

Select the single best response for each question.

20.1   Which of the following is an essential characteristic of infantile autism, as proposed by Rutter (1968)?

  A. Onset before age 30 months.
  B. Bizarre motor behavior.
  C. Impaired language.
  D. Lack of social interest and responsiveness.
  E. All of the above.

The correct response is option E.

Rutter (1968), in his critical analysis of the existing empirical evidence, identified four features present in nearly all children with autism: 1) lack of social interest and responsiveness; 2) impaired language, ranging from absence of speech to peculiar speech patterns; 3) bizarre motor behavior, ranging from rigid and limited play patterns to more complex ritualistic and compulsive behavior; and 4) early onset (before age 30 months). **(p. 261)**

20.2   All of the following are pervasive developmental disorders *except*

  A. Autistic disorder.
  B. Mental retardation.
  C. Rett's disorder.
  D. Childhood disintegrative disorder.
  E. Asperger's disorder.

The correct response is option B.

Mental retardation is not a pervasive developmental disorder. **(p. 262)**

20.3   A common comorbid medical condition noted in patients with autism is epilepsy. Which of the following statements is *true?*

  A. The risk of epilepsy in patients with autism is highest during late adolescence.
  B. A prospective study of epilepsy in children with autistic spectrum disorders found a rate of 5%.
  C. The most common type of epilepsy is generalized or grand mal seizures.
  D. Males with autism have seizures more frequently than do females with autism.
  E. None of the above.

The correct response is option B.

A prospective study of epilepsy in children with autistic spectrum disorder found that about 5% of those with an autistic condition had epilepsy (Wong 1993). The risk of epilepsy in patients with autism seems to be highest in early childhood, not late adolescence. The most common type of seizures are partial seizures, and females have a greater risk of seizures than do males. (p. 267)

20.4 All of the following psychopharmacological agents have been reported to decrease autistic symptoms *except*

A. Fluoxetine.
B. Fluvoxamine.
C. Quetiapine.
D. Venlafaxine.
E. Sertraline.

The correct response is option C.

In an open-label quetiapine treatment trial in six autistic children, Martin et al. (1999) reported that there was no significant improvement as rated on the Clinical Global Impressions Scale. Quetiapine was also poorly tolerated by many patients and was associated with serious side effects. (p. 292)

20.5 Which of the following factors has consistently been shown to be related to outcome in autistic patients?

A. Age at onset.
B. Family history of mental illness.
C. IQ.
D. Perinatal complications.
E. Birth weight.

The correct response is option C.

Three factors have consistently been shown to be related to outcome in autistic patients: IQ, presence or absence of speech, and severity of the disorder. Outcome does not appear to be related to age at onset, family history of mental illness, perinatal complications, or birth weight. (p. 296)

References

Martin A, Koenig K, Scahill L, et al: Open-label quetiapine in the treatment of children and adolescents with autistic disorder. J Child Adolesc Psychopharmacol 9:99–107, 1999

Rutter M: Concepts of autism: a review of research. J Child Psychol Psychiatry 9:1–25, 1968

Wong V: Epilepsy in children with autistic spectrum disorder. J Child Neurol 8:316–322, 1993

C H A P T E R   2 1

Other Pervasive Developmental Disorders

Select the single best response for each question.

21.1   Which of the following symptoms is *least* likely to be present in Asperger's disorder?

    A. Impairment in nonverbal social interactions.
    B. Impairment in peer relationships.
    C. General delay in language development.
    D. Lack of social or emotional reciprocity.
    E. Restricted repetitive or stereotyped patterns of behavior or interests.

The correct response is option C.

There is no clinically significant general delay in language in Asperger's disorder. **(p. 318)**

21.2   In regard to differences between Asperger's disorder and autistic disorder, all of the following clinical and research findings are correct *except*

    A. Asperger's disorder may be associated with a higher verbal IQ than found in high-functioning autism (Klin et al. 1995; Ramberg et al. 1996).
    B. On the Wechsler Intelligence Scale for Children—Revised, individuals with Asperger's disorder had good verbal ability and troughs on Object Assembly and Coding, whereas those with autistic disorder had a peak on Block Design (Ehlers et al. 1997).
    C. On the Rorschach inkblot test, adolescents with Asperger's had lower levels of disorganized thinking than did those with high-functioning autism (Ghaziuddin et al. 1995).
    D. In a study examining the development of theory of mind in children with autism and Asperger's disorder, Asperger patients performed better than autism patients on false belief, belief term comprehension, and belief term expression tasks (Ziatas et al. 1998).
    E. Asperger patients are more likely than autism patients to be argumentative, aggressive, and condescending.

The correct response is option C.

On the Rorschach inkblot test, adolescents with Asperger's disorder were observed as having higher, not lower, levels of disorganized thinking than adolescents with high-functioning autistic disorder (Ghaziuddin et al. 1995). **(p. 320)**

21.3 In Hagberg and Witt-Engerström's (1986) four-stage model of the course of neurological deterioration in Rett's disorder, the *rapid developmental regression stage*

A. Often occurs during school age or early adolescence.
B. Occurs between the ages of 6 months and 1.5 years, with a median age of 10–11 months.
C. Usually occurs at age 1–2 years and lasts for 13–19 months.
D. Usually occurs at age 3–4 years but can be delayed and can persist for many years or even decades.
E. Marks the period of slowest deterioration of all stages.

The correct response is option C.

The *rapid developmental regression stage* usually occurs at age 1–2 years and lasts for 13–19 months. The *early-onset stagnation stage* occurs between the ages of 6 months and 1.5 years, with a median age of 10–11 months. The *pseudostationary stage* usually occurs at age 3–4 years, but it can be delayed and can persist for many years or even decades. The *late motor deterioration stage* often occurs during school age or early adolescence. **(p. 333)**

21.4 Which of the following statements concerning childhood disintegrative disorder is *true*?

A. Childhood disintegrative disorder is a common condition.
B. It usually develops during the first year of life.
C. The developmental regression, once initiated, typically progresses over a period of several years.
D. Children rarely regain any language ability once developmental regression has occurred.
E. It is associated with a high prevalence of epilepsy.

The correct response is option E.

In a study of 13 patients with childhood disintegrative disorder, Mouridsen et al. (1999) found that 77% of the patients had epilepsy, and that in 50%, the epilepsy was of the psychomotor variant. Childhood disintegrative disorder is extremely rare. Individuals with the disorder have normal or near-normal development until the age of 3 or 4 years. After the regression phase, children remain stable for many years. Volkmar (1992) reported that as many as 40% of patients regain the ability to speak in single words, with 20% regaining the capacity to speak in sentences. **(pp. 334–336)**

21.5 The DSM-IV-TR (American Psychiatric Association 2000) subtype *residual autism* of pervasive developmental disorder not otherwise specified (PDDNOS) is exemplified by which of the following?

A. Individuals who "almost but not quite" meet the full criteria for autism.
B. Individuals who have a history of autism but who currently do not meet full criteria.
C. Individuals who "almost but not quite" meet criteria for Asperger's disorder.
D. Individuals who show mixed features of autism and Asperger's disorder.
E. Individuals with comorbid medical or neurological disorders associated with autism.

The correct response is option B.

The PDDNOS subtype *residual autism* describes individuals with a history of autistic disorder who currently do not meet the full criteria for autistic disorder (i.e., who still have some autistic features subsequent to effective interventions and/or natural development). **(p. 338)**

References

American Psychiatric Association: Diagnostic and Statistical Manual of Mental Disorders, 4th Edition, Text Revision. Washington, DC, American Psychiatric Association, 2000

Ehlers S, Nyden A, Gillberg C, et al: Asperger syndrome, autism and attention disorder: a comparative study of cognitive profiles of 120 children. J Child Psychol Psychiatry 38:207–217, 1997

Ghaziuddin M, Leininger L, Tsai L: Brief report: thought disorder in Asperger syndrome: comparison with high-functioning autism. J Autism Dev Disord 25:311–317, 1995

Hagberg B, Witt-Engerström I: Rett syndrome: a suggested staging system for describing impairment profile with increasing age towards adolescence. Am J Med Genet Suppl 1:47–59, 1986

Klin A, Volkmar FR, Sparrow SS, et al: Validity and neuropsychological characterization of Asperger syndrome: convergence with nonverbal learning disabilities syndrome. J Child Psychol Psychiatry 36:1127–1140, 1995

Mouridsen SE, Rich B, Isager T: Epilepsy in disintegrative psychosis and infantile autism: a long-term validation study. Dev Med Child Neurol 41:110–114, 1999

Ramberg C, Ehlers S, Nyden A, et al: Language and pragmatic functions in school-age children on the autism spectrum. Eur J Disord Commun 31:387–413, 1996

Volkmar FR: Childhood disintegrative disorder: issues for DSM-IV. J Autism Dev Disord 22:625–642, 1992

Ziatas K, Durkin K, Pratt C: Belief term development in children with autism, Asperger syndrome, specific language impairment, and normal development: links to theory of mind development. J Child Psychol Psychiatry 39:755–763, 1998

C H A P T E R   2 2

Developmental Disorders of Learning, Motor Skills, and Communication

Select the single best response for each question.

22.1 Which of the following statements concerning the clinical presentation of learning disorders is *false?*

A. Reading disorder occurs in 2%–20% of children.
B. Reading disorder accounts for up to 80% of all children diagnosed with a learning disorder.
C. An equal proportion of boys and girls are diagnosed with a reading disorder.
D. Disorder of written expression is more common in boys than in girls.
E. Mathematics disorder is reported to occur in 1%–6% of school-age children.

The correct response is option C.

Approximately 80% of children diagnosed with a reading disorder are boys (American Psychiatric Association 2000). **(p. 355)**

22.2 All of the following statements concerning developmental coordination disorder are correct *except*

A. The disorder occurs in up to 6% of 5- to 11-year-olds.
B. The clumsiness associated with this disorder can lead to peer teasing.
C. Children with developmental coordination disorder seldom have associated delays of other developmental milestones.
D. Comorbid conditions such as attention-deficit/hyperactivity disorder (ADHD) are frequently seen in children with developmental coordination disorder.
E. The coordination deficits may continue throughout life.

The correct response is option C.

Developmental coordination disorder occurs in up to 6% of 5- to 11-year-olds. It is usually first diagnosed when parents notice a delay in development of specific motor skills, or difficulty with skills once attempted. The disorder often is associated with delays in other developmental milestones, and it may be comorbid with ADHD and other conditions. The clumsiness associated with this disorder often leads to peer teasing, which can have a harmful emotional impact. Although motor deficits can be remediated, in some cases problems continue throughout life. **(p. 360)**

22.3 In language, *morphology* is defined as

A. A language's sound system and accompanying rules governing the combination of sounds.
B. The system that governs the structure and formation of words in a language.
C. The system that governs the order and combination of words to form sentences.
D. The system that governs the meaning of words and sentences.
E. The system that combines the language components into functional and socially appropriate communication.

The correct response is option B.

Morphology is the system that governs the structure and formation of words in a language. *Phonology* is a language's sound system and accompanying rules governing the combination of sounds. *Syntax* is the system that governs the order and combination of words to form sentences. *Semantics* is the system that governs the meaning of words and sentences. *Pragmatics* is the system that combines all of the above language components into functional and socially appropriate communication. **(p. 361, Table 22–7)**

22.4 Which of the following communication disorders disproportionately affects males?

A. Developmental (versus acquired) expressive language disorder.
B. Mixed receptive–expressive language disorder.
C. Phonological disorder.
D. Stuttering.
E. All of the above.

The correct response is option E.

Although there is some evidence that referral bias may contribute to the higher prevalence rates of developmental expressive language disorder and mixed receptive–expressive language disorder in boys, all of the disorders listed above are believed to affect males more often than females. **(p. 364)**

22.5 Which of the following statements concerning the etiology of communication disorders is *false*?

A. The etiology is primarily due to family environment and sociological factors.
B. Exposure to intrauterine teratogens may adversely affect language development.
C. Anoxia and asphyxia have been implicated in the development of communication disorders.
D. Important environmental risk factors for the development of communication disorders include poverty and abuse or neglect.
E. Early childhood risk factors that have been implicated in communication disorders include persistent otitis media and other childhood illnesses.

The correct response is option A.

The etiology of communication disorders is primarily biological, although family environment and sociological factors also play a role. **(p. 367)**

Reference

American Psychiatric Association: Diagnostic and Statistical Manual of Mental Disorders, 4th Edition, Text Revision. Washington, DC, American Psychiatric Association, 2000

CHAPTER 23

Schizophrenia and Other Psychotic Disorders

Select the single best response for each question.

23.1   The diagnosis of schizophrenia with childhood onset

    A. Is a common presentation for this disorder.
    B. Is five times more likely in females than in males.
    C. Requires no mood disorder exclusion.
    D. Can be made when signs of disturbance have been present for at least 3 months.
    E. May have a prevalence of less than 1 in 1,000.

The correct response is option E.

Population studies have suggested that the prevalence of childhood-onset schizophrenia may be less than 1 in 1,000. Spencer and Campbell (1994) reported a male-to-female ratio of 3.8 to 1 in a sample of 24 children. In diagnosing schizophrenia, mood disorders and schizoaffective disorders must be ruled out. The diagnosis can be made when signs of the disturbance have been present for at least 6 months, with at least 1 month of active-phase symptoms. **(p. 380)**

23.2   In regard to National Institute of Mental Health studies comparing patients with childhood-onset schizophrenia and patients with adult-onset schizophrenia, all of the following findings are correct *except*

    A. Childhood-onset patients showed greater delay in language development than did adult-onset patients.
    B. Childhood-onset patients evidenced more disruptive behavior disorders than did adult-onset patients.
    C. Childhood-onset patients evidenced more learning disorders than did adult-onset patients.
    D. Childhood-onset patients evidenced few motor stereotypies.
    E. Childhood-onset schizophrenia appears to represent a more malignant form of the disorder.

The correct response is option D.

Patients with childhood-onset schizophrenia commonly present with motor stereotypies (Alaghband-Rad et al. 1995). **(p. 382)**

23.3   Which phase of illness in schizophrenic patients is best described by the following definition: "A 1- to 6-month (or longer) period when symptoms of hallucinations, delusions, thought disorder, or disorganized behavior are predominant?"

A. Prodrome.
B. Acute phase.
C. Recovery phase.
D. Residual phase.
E. Chronicity.

The correct response is option B.

During the *acute phase*, which usually lasts 1–6 months or longer, positive symptoms (i.e., hallucinations, delusions, thought disorder, and disorganized behavior) are predominant. **(p. 388)**

23.4   Which of the following statements concerning the differential diagnosis of childhood psychotic disorders is *true*?

A. The diagnostic criteria for schizophreniform disorder require an illness duration of less than 6 months.
B. Once a diagnosis of schizophreniform disorder is made, a diagnosis of schizophrenia can never be given.
C. A diagnosis of schizophreniform disorder requires the presence of a decline in function.
D. Brief psychotic disorder requires a symptom duration of at least 1 month but no more than 6 months.
E. The diagnosis of psychotic disorder not otherwise specified is very rare in the hospitalized adolescent population.

The correct response is option A.

To qualify for a schizophreniform disorder diagnosis, a child must have an illness duration of less than 6 months. With time, a child with schizophreniform disorder may warrant a diagnosis of schizophrenia. **(p. 391)**

23.5   Magnetic resonance imaging (MRI) studies in children with schizophrenia have reported all of the following findings *except*

A. Decreases in total cerebral volume.
B. Cerebral asymmetry.
C. Decreases in ventricular volume.
D. Increases in temporal lobe volume.
E. Decreases in midsagittal thalamic area.

The correct response is option C.

MRI studies in children with schizophrenia have reported *increases* in ventricular volume and decreases in total cerebral volume (Rapoport et al. 1997, 1999). Other findings reported in children with childhood-onset schizophrenia were larger volumes of the superior temporal lobe gyrus (Jacobsen et al. 1996) and a smaller midsagittal thalamic area (Frazier et al. 1996). **(p. 396)**

References

Alaghband-Rad J, McKenna K, Gordon CT: Childhood-onset schizophrenia: the severity of premorbid course. J Am Acad Child Adolesc Psychiatry 34:1273–1283, 1995

Frazier JA, Giedd JA, Hamburger SD, et al: Brain anatomic magnetic resonance imaging in childhood-onset schizophrenia. Arch Gen Psychiatry 53:617–624, 1996

Jacobsen LK, Giedd JN, Vaituzis AC, et al: Temporal lobe morphology in childhood-onset schizophrenia. Am J Psychiatry 153:355–361, 1996

Rapoport JL, Giedd J, Kumra S, et al: Childhood-onset schizophrenia. Progressive ventricular change during adolescence. Arch Gen Psychiatry 54:897–903, 1997

Rapoport JL, Giedd JN, Blumenthal J: Progressive cortical change during adolescence in childhood-onset schizophrenia: a longitudinal magnetic resonance imaging study. Arch Gen Psychiatry 56:649–654, 1999

Spencer EK, Campbell M: Children with schizophrenia: diagnosis, phenomenology, and pharmacotherapy. Schizophr Bull 20:713–725, 1994

CHAPTER 24

Mood Disorders in Prepubertal Children

Select the single best response for each question.

24.1 Childhood mood disorders are often underdiagnosed or misdiagnosed for which of the following reasons?

 A. The belief, on the part of some clinicians, that a child's immature superego and personality structure do not permit the development of a mood disorder.
 B. Many children lack the capacity to express their emotions verbally.
 C. Many children present with somatic complaints that are diagnosed as physical illness.
 D. Parents who are bipolar are often underdiagnosed.
 E. All of the above.

The correct response is option E.

All of the reasons above are contributing factors to the underdiagnosis or misdiagnosis of childhood mood disorders. **(p. 411)**

24.2 Prepubertal children with major depression routinely present with atypical features. Symptoms consistent with such a presentation include all of the following *except*

 A. Hypersomnia.
 B. Weight loss.
 C. Psychomotor retardation.
 D. Mood reactivity.
 E. Increased appetite.

The correct response is option B.

Weight *gain* is a more likely presentation in childhood atypical depression. **(pp. 413–414)**

24.3 In contrast to manic adults, manic children usually present with all of the following symptoms *except*

 A. Irritability.
 B. Impulsivity.
 C. Euphoria.
 D. Depression.
 E. Inability to concentrate.

The correct response is option C.

In contrast to manic adults, manic children are seldom characterized by euphoric mood. Instead, the mania in young children usually presents as irritability, aggressive temper outbursts, worsening of disruptive behavior, moodiness, difficulty sleeping at night, impulsivity, hyperactivity, inability to concentrate, explosive anger followed by guilt, depression, and poor school performance. **(p. 415)**

24.4   What proportion of children with major depressive episodes show signs of bipolar disorder by adolescence?

    A. One-quarter.
    B. One-third.
    C. One-half.
    D. Two-thirds.
    E. Three-fourths.

The correct response is option B.

As many as one-third of children with major depressive episodes may show signs of bipolar disorder by adolescence (Geller et al. 1994). **(p. 416)**

24.5   Which of the following statements concerning school-age children with mood disorders is *true*?

    A. They do not attempt suicide.
    B. They are unable to describe their symptoms.
    C. They tend not to somatize their symptoms.
    D. Mania is usually characterized by pressured speech.
    E. School performance is usually unaffected.

The correct response is option D.

Mania in school-age children is characterized by pressured speech that is difficult or impossible to interrupt. **(p. 417)**

Reference

Geller B, Fox LW, Clark KA: Rate and predictors of prepubertal bipolarity during follow-up of 6- to 12-year-old depressed children. J Am Acad Child Adolesc Psychiatry 33:461–468, 1994

C H A P T E R 2 5

Mood Disorders in Adolescents

Select the single best response for each question.

25.1 Commonly presenting symptoms of depression in adolescents include

   A. Poor school performance.
   B. Social withdrawal.
   C. Substance abuse.
   D. Conduct disorder.
   E. All of the above.

The correct response is option E.

Substance abuse is the presenting symptom in approximately 20% of adolescents with mood disorders (Weller and Weller 1990). Poor school performance, social withdrawal, conduct disorder, and promiscuous sexual behavior are also common among depressed adolescents. **(p. 439)**

25.2 Diagnosing bipolar disorder in adolescence may be challenging for all of the following reasons *except*

   A. Presenting symptoms are often minor or major depression.
   B. Severity of symptoms frequently results in hospitalization.
   C. Because symptoms may build up gradually, they frequently are overlooked.
   D. Inappropriate sexual behavior and other "atypical" presentation are common.
   E. Serious conduct behaviors, such as vandalism, may mask underlying manic symptoms.

The correct response is option B.

In adolescents, symptoms frequently do not receive clinical attention because they may build up gradually. McGlashan (1988) noted that a delay of up to 5 years often occurs between the onset of symptoms during adolescence and an episode of sufficient severity to require hospitalization or treatment. **(p. 443)**

25.3 In a study by Carlson et al. (2000) comparing patients with early-onset (between the ages of 15 and 20 years) and adult-onset bipolar disorder, which of the following findings was reported?

   A. Women predominated in the early-onset group.
   B. More remissions occurred during follow-up in the early-onset group than in the adult-onset group.
   C. Individuals in the early-onset group were more likely than those in the adult-onset group to have a substance use disorder.
   D. Patients with early-onset bipolar disorder had an increased risk of mood-incongruent psychotic symptoms.
   E. Depressive episodes occurred more frequently in the early-onset group.

The correct response is option C.

Early-onset bipolar patients were more likely than adult-onset patients to have a substance use disorder at the onset of their bipolar disorder (Carlson et al. 2000). Males predominated in the early-onset group. Mood-incongruent psychotic symptoms were equally likely in early-onset and adult-onset bipolar patients. Fewer remissions were seen in early-onset patients, and manic, not depressive, episodes occurred more frequently in this group. **(pp. 443–444)**

25.4   Approximately 40%–70% of children and adolescents with major depressive disorder have a comorbid psychiatric disorder. All of the following are common comorbid conditions *except*

    A. Eating disorders.
    B. Anxiety disorders.
    C. Dysthymic disorder.
    D. Disruptive behavior disorder.
    E. Substance use.

The correct response is option A.

Eating disorders are not common comorbid conditions in children and adolescents with major depressive disorder. The most frequent comorbid diagnoses are dysthymic disorder (30%–80%), anxiety disorders (30%–80%), disruptive disorders (10%–80%), and substance abuse (20%–30%). Twenty to fifty percent of children with major depressive disorder have two or more comorbid diagnoses. **(pp. 444–445)**

25.5   Common side effects of lithium treatment in children and adolescents include all of the following *except*

    A. Diarrhea.
    B. Tremor.
    C. Leukopenia.
    D. Fatigue.
    E. Ataxia.

The correct response is option C.

Common lithium side effects in youth include nausea, diarrhea, tremor, enuresis, fatigue, ataxia, and leukocytosis (*not* leukopenia). **(p. 465)**

References

Carlson GA, Bromet EJ, Sievers S: Phenomenology and outcome of subjects with early and adult-onset psychotic mania. Am J Psychiatry 157:213–219, 2000

McGlashan TH: Adolescent versus adult onset of mania. Am J Psychiatry 145:221–223, 1988

Weller EB, Weller RA: Depressive disorders in children and adolescents, in Psychiatric Disorders in Children and Adolescents. Edited by Garfinkel BD. Philadelphia, PA, WB Saunders, 1990, pp 3–20

C H A P T E R   2 6

Attention-Deficit/
Hyperactivity Disorder

Select the single best response for each question.

26.1 Which of the following is *not* one of the core symptom clusters of attention-deficit/hyperactivity disorder (ADHD) as identified in DSM-IV-TR (American Psychiatric Association 2000)?

A. Hyperactivity.
B. Inattention.
C. Impulsivity.
D. Disruptive behavior.
E. Distractibility.

The correct response is option D.

Inattention, hyperactivity, and impulsivity are the core symptom clusters in ADHD. Disruptive behavior is not a core symptom of the disorder, although it may be present. **(pp. 485–486)**

26.2 Which of the following is *not* one of the DSM-IV-TR diagnostic criteria for ADHD?

A. Symptoms must have persisted for at least 6 months.
B. Symptoms must be evident in at least two different environments.
C. Symptoms must have been present before age 5 years.
D. Symptoms must be maladaptive in terms of functioning.
E. Symptoms cannot be accounted for by another DSM-IV-TR diagnosis (e.g., a pervasive developmental disorder).

The correct response is option C.

Some symptoms that caused impairment must have been present before age 7 years. **(pp. 486–487, Table 26–1)**

26.3 Which of the following comorbid psychiatric disorders has been reported to occur most frequently in children diagnosed with ADHD?

A. Schizophrenia.
B. Oppositional defiant disorder.
C. Autism.
D. Bipolar disorder.
E. Panic disorder.

The correct response is option B.

Oppositional defiant disorder and conduct disorder occur with a high frequency in children with ADHD (as many as 30%–50%) (Biederman et al. 1991). **(p. 491)**

26.4   Which of the following statements concerning the epidemiology of ADHD is *false?*

A. The disorder seems to be more common in boys than in girls.
B. The prevalence reported in DSM-IV-TR is 3%–7% of school-age children.
C. ADHD is more common in school-age populations than in older populations.
D. Prevalence rates show little variation across cultures, countries, and settings (urban, suburban, and rural).
E. None of the above.

The correct response is option D.

Rates of ADHD may vary across different cultures and countries, as well as according to whether the sample studied is urban, suburban, or rural. **(p. 492)**

26.5   Which of the following statements concerning research findings on the course and duration of ADHD is *correct?*

A. At least some impairment from the disorder is present in most adolescents who were referred for clinical treatment as school-age children.
B. The disorder is generally episodic rather than chronic.
C. Inattention tends to remit over time, in contrast to hyperactivity, which is remarkably persistent.
D. Inattention symptoms may place a child at greater risk for the development of antisocial behavior.
E. None of the above.

The correct response is option A.

Prospective studies of clinical samples report that at least some impairment from the disorder is present in most adolescents who were referred for clinical treatment as school-age children (Barkley et al. 1991; Gittelman et al. 1985). The disorder is generally chronic and enduring (Keller et al. 1992). Inattention problems are remarkably persistent and intractable, whereas hyperactivity tends to remit over time (Biederman et al. 2000). Hyperactivity and impulsivity symptoms may place a child at greater risk for the development of antisocial outcomes (Babinski et al. 1999). **(p. 495)**

26.6   The research literature supports the use of all of the following medications for ADHD *except*

A. Tricyclic antidepressants.
B. Psychostimulants.
C. Clonidine.
D. Bupropion.
E. Benzodiazepines.

The correct response is option E.

Benzodiazepines are not recommended in the treatment of ADHD. Psychostimulants are the agents of choice for symptom suppression. Tricyclic antidepressants are considered second-line agents. Both clonidine and bupropion have shown some promise in the treatment of ADHD symptoms. **(pp. 495–497)**

References

American Psychiatric Association: Diagnostic and Statistical Manual of Mental Disorders, 4th Edition, Text Revision. Washington, DC, American Psychiatric Association, 2000

Babinski LM, Hartsough CS, Lambert NM: Childhood conduct problems, hyperactivity-impulsivity, and inattention as predictors of adult criminal activity. J Child Psychol Psychiatry 40:347–355, 1999

Barkley RA, Fischer M, Edelbrock C, et al: The adolescent outcome of hyperactive children diagnosed by research criteria, III: mother-child interactions, family conflicts and maternal psychopathology. J Child Psychol Psychiatry 32:233–255, 1991

Biederman J, Newcorn J, Sprich S: Comorbidity of attention deficit hyperactivity disorder with conduct, depressive, anxiety, and other disorders. Am J Psychiatry 148:564–577, 1991

Biederman J, Mick E, Faraone SV: Age-dependent decline of symptoms of attention deficit hyperactivity disorder: impact of remission definition and symptom type. Am J Psychiatry 157:816–818, 2000

Gittelman R, Mannuzza S, Shenker R, et al: Hyperactive boys almost grown up, I: psychiatric status. Arch Gen Psychiatry 42:937–947, 1985

Keller MB, Lavori PW, Beardslee WR, et al: The disruptive behavioral disorder in children and adolescents: comorbidity and clinical course. J Am Acad Child Adolesc Psychiatry 31:204–209, 1992

C H A P T E R 2 7

Conduct Disorder and Oppositional Defiant Disorder

Select the single best response for each question.

27.1 Which of the following statements regarding the diagnoses of conduct disorder and oppositional defiant disorder (ODD) is *true?*

A. Children with these disorders are a distinct group that presents in a uniform and narrow fashion.
B. The relationship between conduct disorder and ODD is clearly defined.
C. The diagnosis of conduct disorder is controversial in child psychiatry.
D. ODD behaviors typically are preceded by more serious violations of age-appropriate behavioral norms.
E. Conduct disorder has been determined to be a biological condition.

The correct response is option C.

The classification of conduct disorder is a controversial and unsettled issue in mental health. Children with conduct disorder represent a varied group because of the myriad of manifestations of antisocial behavior and the complex factors that contribute to it. The relationship between conduct disorder and ODD remains unclear. ODD behaviors tend to precede more serious violations of age-appropriate behavioral norms. The etiology of conduct disorder is manifold, with biological, psychological, and social factors all playing a role. **(p. 509)**

27.2 All of the following statements regarding the prevalence of conduct disorder are correct *except*

A. The prevalence of conduct disorder is difficult to estimate because of variations in definition.
B. The prevalence is estimated as approximately 9% for males and 2% for females younger than 18 years.
C. The childhood-onset type of the disorder (onset before 10 years of age) is clearly much more common in males.
D. Individuals with adolescent-onset conduct disorder are much more likely to develop adult antisocial personality disorder than are those with childhood-onset conduct disorder.
E. Adolescent-onset conduct disorder is less likely than childhood-onset conduct disorder to involve a preponderance of males.

The correct response is option D.

Individuals with childhood-onset conduct disorder are more likely than those with adolescent-onset conduct disorder to develop antisocial personality disorder. **(pp. 509–510)**

27.3 Which of the following statements regarding subtypes of conduct disorder is *true?*

A. Subtyping aggressive behavior into predatory and affective categories is not a useful distinction.
B. Predatory aggression is characterized by the presence of high levels of autonomic and emotional arousal with little apparent instrumental gain.
C. Children who demonstrate reactive aggression tend to be more delinquent than those demonstrating proactive aggression.
D. The process of subclassifying conduct disorder according to age at onset, degree of aggressivity, and extent of socialization has been completely validated.
E. The value of subtyping conduct disorder into childhood-onset and adolescent-onset variants is related to the prognostic significance of age at onset.

The correct response is option E.

The value of subtyping conduct disorder into childhood-onset and adolescent-onset is clearly related to the prognostic significance of age at onset, with early onset being more ominous. Subtyping aggressive behavior into predatory and affective categories is a useful distinction. Predatory aggression is goal directed and involves minimal associated autonomic arousal. Affective aggression is characterized by the presence of high levels of autonomic and emotional arousal with little apparent instrumental gain. Children who manifest proactive aggression are more delinquent that those demonstrating reactive aggression. No system of subtyping conduct disorder has been completely validated. **(pp. 510–511)**

27.4 A biological factor associated with conduct disorder is

A. Reduced novelty-seeking trait.
B. A history of maternal smoking during pregnancy.
C. Anxious temperament.
D. Reduced rates of expression of the L/L variant of the serotonin transporter gene.
E. Elevated harm-avoidance trait.

The correct response is option B.

Wakschlag et al. (1997) demonstrated that maternal smoking during pregnancy was associated with a significant increase in the rate of conduct disorder, even after adjustment for previously identified risk factors. Adolescents who showed elevations in novelty seeking and reductions in harm avoidance demonstrated increased rates of aggressive and delinquent behavior (Schmeck and Poustka 2001). Enhanced rates of expression of the L/L variant of the serotonin transporter gene were found in a sample of hyperactive children and adolescents both with and without conduct disorder (Seeger et al. 2001). **(pp. 513–515)**

27.5 All of the following statements concerning treatment of youngsters with conduct disorder are correct *except*

A. Treatment may take place in a variety of different long-term and short-term programs in outpatient, inpatient, and residential settings.
B. Cognitive-behavioral approaches include improvement in problem-solving skills, impulse control, and anger management.
C. Family therapy is not an effective treatment modality in conduct disorder patients.
D. Parent management training focuses on modifying coercive parent–child interactions that encourage child antisocial behaviors.
E. When used, pharmacotherapy commonly targets aggression in the conduct disorder population.

The correct response is option C.

Tolan et al. (1986), in an extensive literature review, found that family therapy was in many cases more effective than other therapeutic modalities. **(pp. 518–519)**

References

Schmeck K, Poustka F: Temperament and disruptive behavior disorders. Psychopathology 34:159–163, 2001

Seeger G, Schloss P, Schmidt MH: Functional polymorphism within the promoter of the serotonin transporter gene is associated with severe hyperkinetic disorders. Mol Psychiatry 6:235–238, 2001

Tolan PH, Cromwell RE, Brasswell M: Family therapy with delinquents: a critical review of the literature. Fam Process 25:619–650, 1986

Wakschlag LS, Lahey B, Loeber R, et al: Maternal smoking during pregnancy and the risk of conduct disorder in boys. Arch Gen Psychiatry 54:670–676, 1997

C H A P T E R   2 8

Conduct and Antisocial Disorders in Adolescence

Select the single best response for each question.

28.1   Which of the following statements concerning the diagnosis of conduct disorder is *false*?

A. The DSM-IV (American Psychiatric Association 1994) definition of conduct disorder is similar to that found in DSM-III-R (American Psychiatric Association 1987).
B. The child must have manifested five or more of a list of undesirable behaviors in the previous 6 months.
C. A list of 15 undesirable behaviors is grouped into four categories.
D. All of the undesirable behaviors defining conduct disorders occur as part of many other diagnoses.
E. A study of youth from U.S. communities (Lahey et al. 1999) documented a strong association between very early behavior problems and subsequent serious aggressive behaviors.

The correct response is option B.

The child must manifest three or more of the undesirable behaviors in the previous 12 months, with at least one behavior present in the previous 6 months. **(pp. 530–531)**

28.2   Which of the following statements concerning the clinical presentation of conduct and antisocial disorders in adolescent is *true*?

A. Mania in adolescence can mimic attention-deficit/hyperactivity disorder (ADHD), oppositional defiant disorder, and conduct disorder.
B. Studies of adult psychiatric patients as well as studies of psychopathology in violent delinquent adolescents demonstrate little relationship between violence and serious psychopathology.
C. Fewer than 20% of arrested male juveniles have drugs or alcohol in their bloodstreams.
D. ADHD was rarely found to coexist in most cases of early-onset conduct disorder.
E. Less than 25% of children with ADHD also manifest evidence of oppositional defiant disorder or conduct disorder.

The correct response is option A.

Mania in adolescence can mimic ADHD, oppositional defiant disorder, and conduct disorder and does not necessarily have the classic adult presentation. Studies of adult psychiatric patients as well as studies of psychopathology in violent delinquent adolescents indicate that violence and serious psychopathology often go hand in hand. Between 40% and 60% of arrested male juveniles have drugs or alcohol in their bloodstream. ADHD has been reported to coexist in most cases of early-onset conduct disorder. Between 50% and 80% of children with ADHD also manifest evidence of oppositional defiant disorder or conduct disorder. **(pp. 532–534)**

28.3   In animal studies, which chemical has been reported to be of importance in the development of normal bonding?

A. Glutamate.
B. Oxytocin.
C. Progesterone.
D. Gamma-aminobutyric acid (GABA).
E. Estrogen.

The correct response is option B.

Animal studies have shown the importance of oxytocin and vasopressin for normal bonding to occur in certain rodents. Oxytocin has been found to be important in numerous social behaviors. In abused children and adolescents with conduct disorder, the apparent lack of empathy may be the result of early compromise to the limbic-hypothalamic-pituitary-adrenal system and of the biochemical effects of poor nurturing on the developing brain. **(p. 540)**

28.4   According to Kazdin (2001), treatment modalities found to produce positive behavioral change in children with conduct disorder include all of the following *except*

A. Parent management training.
B. Group therapy.
C. Cognitive problem-solving skills training.
D. Multisystemic therapy.
E. Functional family therapy.

The correct response is option B.

Only four kinds of treatments have been validated as producing positive behavioral change: parent management training, cognitive problem-solving skills training, multisystemic therapy, and functional family therapy (Kazdin 2001). **(pp. 544–545)**

28.5   Which of the following statements concerning children who have been diagnosed with conduct disorder is *true*?

A. A majority go on to commit aggressive antisocial acts in adulthood.
B. The overall adult adjustment is often good.
C. Suicide and other forms of violent death are common.
D. Many go on to stable marriages after they outgrow symptoms.
E. Most have satisfactory job histories.

The correct response is option C.

The diagnosis of conduct disorder has a grim prognosis: suicide and other forms of violent death are common outcomes. A minority, not a majority, go on to commit aggressive antisocial acts in adulthood. However, the overall adult adjustment is often poor, as reflected in unstable marriages, unsatisfactory job histories, and the presence of many symptoms of maladaptation other than antisocial behaviors. **(p. 545)**

References

American Psychiatric Association: Diagnostic and Statistical Manual of Mental Disorders, 3rd Edition, Revised. Washington, DC, American Psychiatric Association, 1987

American Psychiatric Association: Diagnostic and Statistical Manual of Mental Disorders, 4th Edition. Washington, DC, American Psychiatric Association, 1994

Kazdin AE: Treatment of conduct disorders, in Conduct Disorders in Childhood and Adolescence (Cambridge Child and Adolescent Psychiatry Series). Edited by Hill J, Maughan B. New York, Cambridge University Press, 2001, pp 408–448

Lahey BB, Goodman SH, Waldman ID, et al: Relation of age of onset to the type and severity of child and adolescent conduct problems. J Abnorm Child Psychol 27:247–260, 1999

C H A P T E R 2 9

Separation Anxiety Disorder and Generalized Anxiety Disorder

Select the single best response for each question.

29.1 Separation anxiety

A. Begins at age 18 months and peaks at age 30 months.
B. Is a normative part of development.
C. Usually indicates the presence of a disorder.
D. Symptoms are seldom subclinically present in the pediatric population.
E. Is rarely persistent and excessive.

The correct response is option B.

Separation anxiety is a normative part of development, typically beginning at around 6–7 months, peaking around 18 months, and decreasing after 30 months. Isolated subclinical separation anxiety disorder (SAD) symptoms can be reasonably common. When separation anxiety is persistent and excessive, a diagnosis of SAD should be considered. **(p. 557)**

29.2 Which of the following DSM-IV-TR (American Psychiatric Association 2000) criteria is *not* required in order to make a diagnosis of generalized anxiety disorder (GAD) in children?

A. Excessive anxiety and worry for at least a 6-month period.
B. Difficulty controlling the worry.
C. Three or more associated physiological symptoms (restlessness, fatigue, difficulty concentrating, irritability, muscle tension, or sleep disturbance).
D. The focus of the worry is not related to another Axis I condition.
E. Presence of clinically significant distress or impairment.

The correct response is option C.

Only one physiological symptom is required for the GAD diagnosis in children, in contrast to the three or more that are required in adults. **(p. 559)**

29.3 Which of the following statements regarding the epidemiology of GAD and SAD is *true*?

A. SAD is more prevalent among older children.
B. GAD is more prevalent among younger children.
C. Rates of SAD increase with age.
D. Rates of SAD and GAD do not vary with age.
E. Rates of GAD increase with age.

The correct response is option E.

Rates of GAD increase with age. SAD is more prevalent among younger children, GAD is more prevalent among older children. Rates of SAD decrease with age, whereas rates of SAD and GAD vary by age. **(p. 561)**

29.4   Which of the following statements about temperament and its contributing role to childhood anxiety is *false?*

    A. Approximately 20% of healthy infants are born with traits that predispose them to become highly reactive in novel environments (Kagan and Snidman 1999).

    B. Kagan (1994) described the temperamental characteristic of behavioral inhibition as a child's tendency to approach unfamiliar or novel situations with distress, restraint, or avoidance.

    C. Behavioral inhibition appears to be a highly unstable temperamental trait.

    D. Children with behavioral inhibition may be differentiated from non–behaviorally inhibited children through neurophysiological markers (Kagan et al. 1988).

    E. Children who are identified as shy may be more prone to anxiety symptoms than those who are not (Biederman et al. 1995).

The correct response is option C.

The tendency to approach or avoid new situations is often an enduring temperamental trait. **(pp. 561–562)**

29.5   The use of selective serotonin reuptake inhibitors (SSRIs) in the treatment of childhood anxiety disorders

    A. Is considered a second-line choice (after benzodiazepines).

    B. Has been supported by the results of several recent randomized, placebo-controlled trials.

    C. Should usually continue indefinitely once initiated.

    D. Has resulted in no documented side effects.

    E. Has resulted in minimal clinical benefit over placebo.

The correct response is option B.

SSRIs are the first-line choice in the pharmacological treatment of childhood anxiety disorders, a conclusion supported by the results of three recent, randomized trials. After remission of target symptoms with SSRIs, a drug-free trial should be considered (Pine 2002). If a youth relapses during the period without medication, the SSRI should be restarted. Stomachaches and increased motor activity have been reported with the use of fluvoxamine (Research Unit on Pediatric Psychopharmacology Anxiety Study Group 2001). Children receiving fluvoxamine (or SSRIs in general) showed a significant decrease in clinician-rated anxiety, compared with the placebo group. **(pp. 564–565)**

References

American Psychiatric Association: Diagnostic and Statistical Manual of Mental Disorders, 4th Edition, Text Revision. Washington, DC, American Psychiatric Association, 2000

Biederman J, Rosenbaum JF, Chaloff J, et al: Behavioral inhibition as a risk factor for anxiety disorders, in Anxiety Disorders in Children and Adolescents. Edited by March JS. New York, Guilford, 1995, pp 61–81

Kagan J: Galen's Prophecy. New York, Basic Books, 1994

Kagan J, Snidman N: Early childhood predictors of adult anxiety disorders. Biol Psychiatry 46:1536–1541, 1999

Kagan J, Reznick JS, Snidman N: Biological bases of childhood shyness. Science 240:167–171, 1988

Pine DS: Treating children and adolescents with selective serotonin reuptake inhibitors: how long is appropriate? J Child Adolesc Psychopharmacol 12:189–203, 2002

Research Unit on Pediatric Psychopharmacology Anxiety Study Group: Fluvoxamine for the treatment of anxiety disorders in children and adolescents. N Engl J Med 344:1279–1285, 2001

CHAPTER 30

Obsessive-Compulsive Disorder

Select the single best response for each question.

30.1   According to studies conducted by Geller et al. (1998) and Swedo et al. (1989), which of the following epidemiological findings related to obsessive-compulsive disorder (OCD) is *false?*

A. Girls tended to have an earlier age at onset.
B. In young children, there was a male predominance (male-to-female ratio: 3 to 2).
C. The mean age at onset was 10 years.
D. Children with early-onset OCD were more likely to have a family member with OCD.
E. In adolescence, the gender distribution between girls and boys with OCD was about equal.

The correct response is option A.

Boys tended to have an earlier age at onset, around age 9 years, whereas girls were more likely to have an onset around puberty, at about age 11 years (Swedo et al. 1989). **(p. 576)**

30.2   Which of the following is *not* a proposed subtype of OCD in children?

A. Early-onset OCD.
B. Late-onset OCD.
C. Tic-related OCD.
D. Streptococcal-precipitated OCD.
E. None of the above.

The correct response is option B.

Late-onset OCD is not a proposed subtype of the disorder in children. **(pp. 577–578)**

30.3   Several lines of neuroscience research have implicated, as a cause for OCD, a dysfunction in which brain structure?

A. Hippocampus.
B. Amygdala.
C. Basal ganglia.
D. Dorsal lateral prefrontal cortex.
E. Substantia nigra.

The correct response is option C.

Several lines of research suggest that OCD may be the result of frontal lobe–limbic–basal ganglia dysfunction. Brain insults that result in basal ganglia damage (e.g., head injury, brain tumors) have been reported to be related to the onset of OCD. **(p. 579)**

30.4   Recent research supports the addition of which of the following pharmacological agents as an appropriate augmentation to a selective serotonin reuptake inhibitor (SSRI)?

   A. Lithium.
   B. Imipramine.
   C. Lamotrigine.
   D. Bupropion.
   E. Risperidone.

The correct response is option E.

A controlled trial of SSRI augmentation (McDougle et al. 2000) demonstrated that the addition of risperidone was superior to placebo in reducing OCD symptoms. **(p. 582)**

30.5   In the largest and most recent systematic follow-up study of children with OCD being treated with SSRIs and behavior therapy (Leonard et al. 1993), what percentage still met diagnostic criteria for OCD 2–7 years after initial presentation?

   A. 17%.
   B. 28%.
   C. 43%.
   D. 68%.
   E. 82%.

The correct response is option C.

Leonard et al. (1993) found that among patients seen 2–7 years after initial presentation, 43% still met diagnostic criteria for OCD. **(p. 584)**

References

Geller DA, Biederman J, Jones J, et al: Is juvenile obsessive-compulsive disorder a developmental subtype of the disorder? a review of the pediatric literature. J Am Acad Child Adolesc Psychiatry 37:420–427, 1998

Leonard HL, Swedo SE, Lenane MC, et al: A 2- to 7-year follow-up study of 54 obsessive compulsive children and adolescents. Arch Gen Psychiatry 50:429–439, 1993

McDougle CJ, Epperson CN, Pelton GH, et al: A double-blind, placebo-controlled study of risperidone addition in serotonin reuptake inhibitor-refractory obsessive-compulsive disorder. Arch Gen Psychiatry 57:794–801, 2000

Swedo S, Rapoport JL, Leonard HL, et al: Obsessive-compulsive disorder in children and adolescents: clinical phenomenology of 70 consecutive cases. Arch Gen Psychiatry 46:335–341, 1989

C H A P T E R   3 1

Specific Phobia, Panic Disorder, Social Phobia, and Selective Mutism

Select the single best response for each question.

31.1 To which of the following disorders does the DSM-IV-TR (American Psychiatric Association 2000) definition "a marked and persistent fear that is excessive or unreasonable, cued by the presence or anticipation of a specific object or situation" apply?

  A. Social phobia.
  B. Selective mutism.
  C. Specific phobia.
  D. Panic disorder.
  E. Anxiety disorder not otherwise specified.

The correct response is option C.

Specific phobia is a marked and persistent fear of circumscribed objects or situations that is excessive or unreasonable. *Social phobia* is a persistent fear of one or more social situations in which a person is exposed to unfamiliar persons or to scrutiny by others. *Selective mutism* is characterized by persistent failure to speak in one or more social situations in which speaking is expected. *Panic disorder* is characterized by recurrent, unexpected panic attacks, which are discrete periods of intense fear or discomfort. **(p. 589)**

31.2 All of the following statements regarding panic disorder are correct *except*

  A. Panic attacks are the hallmark of panic disorder.
  B. Panic disorder may occur with or without agoraphobia.
  C. Children with early development of separation anxiety disorder are at increased risk of later developing panic disorder.
  D. Symptoms, course of illness, and associated complicating conditions in children with panic disorder are very different from those in adults with panic disorder.
  E. Panic disorder may develop at any age during childhood or later.

The correct response is option D.

The symptoms, course, and associated complications and comorbid conditions (agoraphobia, depression) in children and adolescents with panic disorder appear to be very similar to those observed in adults with panic disorder. **(pp. 590, 593)**

31.3   Individuals with social phobia commonly fear which of the following social situations?

A. Public speaking or performing.
B. Attending social gatherings.
C. Dealing with authorities.
D. Asking for directions.
E. All of the above.

The correct response is option E.

Individuals with social phobia fear all of the situations listed above. **(p. 595)**

31.4   In regard to the prevalence of selective mutism in children, which of the following statements is *true?*

A. Prevalence estimates in children range from 3% to 5%.
B. Selective mutism symptoms that occur upon starting school are likely to be unremitting.
C. Variability in prevalence estimates may be due to vagueness in the DSM regarding the level of impairment required to meet diagnostic criteria.
D. Scandinavian prevalence studies have reported lower rates of selective mutism than have U.S. studies among school-age children.
E. Variability in prevalence estimates is unlikely to be related to differences in the consistent application of diagnostic criteria in study populations.

The correct response is option C.

Variability in prevalence estimates may be a function of the age of the children sampled, differences in the application of the diagnostic criteria, and vagueness of the DSM criteria in terms of the degree of impairment required for the diagnosis. **(p. 598)**

31.5   Which of the following descriptions refers to a *top-down* family genetic study of anxiety disorders?

A. The evaluation of the prevalence of anxiety disorders in the offspring of adult probands.
B. The evaluation of the prevalence of anxiety disorders in adult relatives of child probands.
C. The longitudinal evaluation of young offspring of adult probands with anxiety disorders.
D. The comparison of rates of co-occurrence of anxiety disorders in monozygotic twins.
E. The comparison of rates of co-occurrence of anxiety disorders in dizygotic twins.

The correct response is option A.

A *top-down* family genetic study evaluates the prevalence of anxiety disorders in the offspring of adult probands. A *bottom-up* study evaluates the prevalence of anxiety disorders in adult relatives of child and adolescent probands. A *high-risk* study examines young offspring of adult probands with anxiety disorders. A *twin* study compares the rates of co-occurrence of anxiety disorders in monozygotic and dizygotic twin pairs. **(pp. 598–599)**

Reference

American Psychiatric Association: Diagnostic and Statistical Manual of Mental Disorders, 4th Edition, Text Revision. Washington, DC, American Psychiatric Association, 2000

CHAPTER 32

Pediatric Posttraumatic Stress Disorder

Select the single best response for each question.

32.1   In assessing a child for posttraumatic stress disorder (PTSD), clinicians should do all of the following *except*

     A. Establish that the incident actually occurred.
     B. Take children's self-reports of trauma at face value.
     C. Supplement children's self-reports with histories from parents and others.
     D. Remember that children's recollections may be influenced by others.
     E. Use a neutral questioning stance.

The correct response is option B.

Children's self-reports of trauma cannot be taken at face value, because it is known that children may retain false details of their recollection of real trauma. **(pp. 610–612)**

32.2   Stimuli directly or indirectly related to a traumatic event that provoke conditioned responses are known as

     A. Traumatic dreams.
     B. Reenactment behavior.
     C. Traumatic play.
     D. Traumatic reminders.
     E. None of the above.

The correct response is option D.

Traumatic reminders, also called trauma triggers, are stimuli that provoke conditioned responses directly or indirectly related to the traumatic event. *Traumatic dreams* depict personal threats and they renew emotions associated with the experience. *Reenactment behavior* refers to the replication of some aspects of the traumatic experience. *Traumatic play* refers to the repetitive dramatization in play of elements or themes of the event. **(p. 614)**

32.3   Traumatized children frequently have symptoms of disorders other than PTSD. In addition to true comorbidity, spurious comorbidity with PTSD can result from 1) overlap between criteria sets and 2) confounding similar symptoms of other diagnoses with those of PTSD. Which of the following disorders overlaps with or has symptoms similar to those of PTSD?

   A. Attention-deficit/hyperactivity disorder (ADHD).
   B. Oppositional defiant disorder.
   C. Major depressive disorder.
   D. Generalized anxiety disorder.
   E. All of the above.

The correct response is option E.

All of the disorders above have symptoms that overlap with those of PTSD. **(p. 619)**

32.4   Important principles in the psychotherapeutic treatment of children with PTSD include all of the following *except*

   A. Reexposing the individual to traumatic cues under safe conditions.
   B. Allowing the sessions to be unfocused so that unconscious material may be uncovered.
   C. Keeping focused on the child's current dysfunction.
   D. Being diligent about continually rethinking the symptom picture.
   E. Directing the therapy to facilitate higher levels of adaptation and coping.

The correct response is option B.

Psychotherapeutic treatment of children with PTSD should incorporate reparative and mastery elements in a structured, supportive manner. **(p. 625)**

32.5   Which of the following antidepressants has been approved by the U.S. Food and Drug Administration (FDA) for the treatment of PTSD in adults and is often used to treat PTSD in children and adolescents?

   A. Bupropion.
   B. Nefazodone.
   C. Imipramine.
   D. Duloxetine.
   E. Paroxetine.

The correct response is option E.

Paroxetine has received FDA approval for the treatment of PTSD in adults, and it is also often used in children and adolescents. **(p. 628)**

CHAPTER 33

Feeding and Eating Disorders of Infancy and Early Childhood

Select the single best response for each question.

33.1 All of the following statements concerning feeding disorders in infants are correct *except*

   A. Up to 25% of otherwise healthy infants and young children have feeding problems.
   B. Common feeding difficulties include eating too little or too much food, food refusal, restricted food preferences, and bizarre food habits.
   C. Severe feeding problems, such as refusal to eat or vomiting, have been reported to occur in 5%–10% of infants younger than 1 year of age.
   D. Very few studies have followed the natural history of feeding problems.
   E. Up to 80% of infants and young children with developmental handicaps have feeding problems.

The correct response is option C.

Severe feeding problems such as refusal to eat or vomiting (which are associated with poor weight gain) have been reported to occur in only 1%–2% of infants younger than 1 year of age. **(p. 639)**

33.2 *Failure to thrive*

   A. Is an uncommon problem in pediatrics.
   B. Is a term used to describe infants and young children who develop poor attachments to caregivers during infancy.
   C. Was initially researched as a dichotomous condition, differentiated as organic and nonorganic failure to thrive.
   D. Is diagnosed when a child's decelerated or arrested growth results in height and weight below the 25th percentile.
   E. Has a presentation strikingly different from that of the *hospitalism* syndrome of Rene Spitz.

The correct response is option C.

Failure to thrive was initially researched as a dichotomous condition, differentiating between organic and nonorganic failure to thrive. Failure to thrive is a common problem in pediatrics. The term is used to describe infants and young children who have failure in physical growth. Diagnosis is made when the child's decelerated or arrested growth results in weight and height measurements that fall below the fifth percentile on the Boston Growth Standards. The syndrome Rene Spitz (1945) described as *hospitalism* has a presentation similar to that of failure to thrive. **(p. 639)**

33.3 The DSM-IV-TR (American Psychiatric Association 2000) diagnostic criteria for infantile anorexia include which of the following?

A. The child's refusal to eat adequate amounts of food is of at least 1 month's duration.
B. The onset of the food refusal occurs before 6 years of age.
C. The infant communicates hunger signals and evidences interest in food but shows little interest in exploration and/or interaction with the caregiver.
D. The infant shows little growth deficiency.
E. The food refusal may follow a traumatic event.

The correct response is option A.

The diagnostic criteria for infantile anorexia include refusal to eat adequate amounts of food for at least 1 month; onset of the food refusal before age 3 years; failure to communicate hunger signals and to show interest in food, despite showing interest in exploration and interactions with the provider; and presence of significant growth deficiency. In addition, the food refusal must not follow a traumatic event and must not be due to an underlying medical condition. **(p. 644, Table 33–4)**

33.4 All of the following statements regarding posttraumatic feeding disorder are correct *except*

A. Posttraumatic feeding disorder can occur at any age of development, from infancy to adulthood.
B. The disorder is characterized by the sudden onset of total or partial food refusal.
C. The condition has been reported in children who have undergone intubation or the insertion of nasogastric feeding tubes.
D. Some children may refuse liquids but eat solids.
E. Despite food refusal, feeding tends to be an apathetic process, with the child demonstrating neither emotional excitement nor emotional distress.

The correct response is option E.

Feeding appears to be associated with pain or distress, causing anticipatory fear as demonstrated by crying, gagging, or vomiting at the sight of objects associated with feeding. **(p. 649)**

33.5 Which of the following statements regarding the condition *pica* is *true*?

A. The diagnosis requires that a child demonstrate persistent eating of nonnutritive substances for a period of at least 6 months.
B. The diagnosis would be appropriate in a 6-month-old child who often mouths nonnutritive objects.
C. The diagnosis should be made when the ingestion is considered appropriate to the developmental level.
D. Young children with pica often eat paint, plaster, paper, strings, hair, and cloth.
E. Lead poison is no longer considered a common complication to pica.

The correct response is option D.

Young children with pica typically eat paint, plaster, paper, strings, hair, and cloth. The diagnosis requires that a child demonstrate persistent eating of nonnutritive substances for a period of at least 1 month. The eating of nonnutritive substances must be inappropriate to the developmental level. Before ages 18–24 months, mouthing and occasionally eating nonnutritive substances are relatively common. Lead poisoning is the most common complication associated with pica. **(p. 652)**

References

American Psychiatric Association: Diagnostic and Statistical Manual of Mental Disorders, 4th Edition, Text Revision. Washington, DC, American Psychiatric Association, 2000

Spitz R: Hospitalism: an inquiry into the psychiatric conditions of early childhood. Psychoanal Study Child 1:53–74, 1945

C H A P T E R 3 4

Infant and Childhood Obesity

Select the single best response for each question.

34.1 The prevalence of obesity in early childhood is not nearly as well studied as the prevalence of obesity in adulthood. However, the few studies that have been conducted indicate the prevalence of obesity in preschool children to be in the range of

A. 0–5%.
B. 5%–10%.
C. 10%–15%.
D. 15%–20%.
E. 20%–25%.

The correct response is option B.

The prevalence of obesity in preschool-age children has been found to be in the 5%–10% range (Maloney and Klykylo 1983). **(p. 661)**

34.2 According to a report by the Centers for Disease Control and Prevention (2002), the prevalence of obesity in children between the ages of 6 and 19 years is in the range of

A. 2%–5%.
B. 6%–8%.
C. 13%–14%.
D. 21%–23%.
E. 30%–33%.

The correct response is option C.

The report by the Centers for Disease Control and Prevention (2002) estimated the proportion of overweight children (ages 6–11 years) at 13%, and of overweight adolescents (ages 12–19 years) at 14%. **(p. 661)**

34.3 According to the American Academy of Child and Adolescent Psychiatry (1997), if one parent is obese, children have what percentage chance of being obese?

A. 10%.
B. 30%.
C. 40%.
D. 50%.
E. 70%.

The correct response is option D.

If one parent is obese, there is a 50% chance that the children will also be obese, and when both parents are obese, the children have an 80% chance of also being obese (American Academy of Child and Adolescent Psychiatry 1997). **(p. 662)**

34.4 Which of the following statements concerning the genetic/familial form of obesity is *true*?

A. There is evidence of psychopathology in the child or parent.
B. Evidence of nutritional misinformation is seen.
C. The family history for obesity is negative.
D. The obesity has a sudden onset, usually around ages 12–13 years.
E. The child may have characteristics associated with "difficult temperament."

The correct response is option E.

In genetic/familial obesity, the child may have characteristics associated with the so-called difficult temperament (low rhythm/predictability and low persistence/attention). In this form of obesity, there is no evidence of psychopathology or nutritional misinformation, but the family history of obesity is positive. Usually the obesity is gradual and progressive, starting by age 5 or 6 years. **(p. 664)**

34.5 Which of the following statements regarding psychogenic obesity is *true*?

A. There is evidence of psychopathology in the child or parent.
B. There is no evidence of nutritional misinformation.
C. The family history for obesity is negative.
D. In one type, associated with traumatic separation from the primary caregiver, there is a sudden onset, usually before age 3 years.
E. All of the above.

The correct response is option E.

All of the statements above characterize psychogenic obesity. **(p. 664)**

References

American Academy of Child and Adolescent Psychiatry: Obesity in children and teens. Facts for Families Series (79). Washington, DC, American Academy of Child and Adolescent Psychiatry, 1997. Available at: http://www.aacap.org/publications/factsfam/79.htm. Accessed May 4, 2003.

Centers for Disease Control and Prevention: Prevalence of overweight among children and adolescents: United States, 1999. Hyattsville, MD, National Center for Health Statistics, 2002

Maloney MJ, Klykylo WM: An overview of anorexia nervosa, bulimia, and obesity in children and adolescents. J Am Acad Child Psychiatry 22:99–107, 1983

CHAPTER 35

Anorexia Nervosa

Select the single best response for each question.

35.1 The DSM-IV-TR (American Psychiatric Association 2000) diagnostic criteria for anorexia nervosa include which of the following?

   A. Body weight less than 50% of that expected.
   B. Body height less than 85% of that expected.
   C. Apathy to weight change.
   D. Amenorrhea in postmenarcheal females.
   E. Loss of interest in body habitus.

The correct response is option D.

Amenorrhea is present in postmenarcheal females afflicted by anorexia nervosa. Patients refuse to maintain body weight at or above a minimally normal weight for age and height; they have an intense fear of gaining weight, deny the seriousness of their current low body weight, and place undue value on body weight and shape on self-evaluation. **(p. 672)**

35.2 DSM-IV-TR distinguishes between two subtypes of anorexia nervosa. Which of the following statements regarding these subtypes is *false?*

   A. The two subtypes are restricting and binge-eating/purging anorexia.
   B. Those with restricting anorexia are more likely to have drug use disorders.
   C. Those with binge-eating/purging anorexia are more likely to display impulse-control problems and mood lability.
   D. Those with binge-eating/purging anorexia score higher on the Psychopathic Deviate, Depression, and Psychasthenia scales of the Minnesota Multiphasic Personality Inventory.
   E. The majority of patients with restricting anorexia develop bulimic symptoms during the course of the disorder.

The correct response is option B.

Patients with restricting anorexia are less likely those with binge-eating/purging anorexia to have drug use disorders. **(pp. 671–672)**

35.3 Common signs and symptoms associated with anorexia nervosa include which of the following?

   A. Heat intolerance.
   B. Tachycardia.
   C. Diarrhea.
   D. Breast engorgement.
   E. Growth of lanugo hair.

The correct response is option E.

Common signs and symptoms of anorexia nervosa include growth of lanugo hair; cold intolerance; bradycardia; constipation; breast atrophy; dental enamel erosion; lesions on the dorsal surfaces of the hands, known as Russell's sign; and dry and yellow-tinged skin. **(p. 672)**

35.4   Which of the following medical complications is *not* routinely associated with anorexia nervosa?

   A. Arrhythmias.
   B. Leukopenia.
   C. Neurological abnormalities.
   D. Decreased gastric motility.
   E. Decreased bone mineral density.

The correct response is option C.

Neurological abnormalities are rarely found in physical examination of patients with anorexia nervosa. Electrocardiographic abnormalities, mild anemia and leukopenia, decreased gastric motility, and delayed gastric emptying are commonly found in anorexic patients. Bone mineral density is reduced at several skeletal sites in most women with anorexia nervosa. **(p. 673)**

35.5   Which of the following statements regarding the use of pharmacotherapy in the treatment of anorexia nervosa is *true*?

   A. Medication has no adjunctive role.
   B. Many psychotropic medications have been shown to effectively reverse the disorder.
   C. Clomipramine and lithium have shown positive effects in clinical studies.
   D. Fluoxetine may have a role in maintaining weight in weight-recovered anorexia patients.
   E. Pharmacotherapy has been shown to be superior to combined medication–psychotherapy treatment in several studies.

The correct response is option D.

Fluoxetine has shown promise in the treatment of weight-recovered anorexic patients. Pharmacotherapy can be a useful adjunct to other treatments. To date, no psychotropic medication has been demonstrated to effectively reverse anorexia nervosa. Clomipramine and lithium have yielded negative or equivocal results in clinical studies. Psychotropic medication should be used only in the context of psychotherapy. **(pp. 683–684)**

Reference

American Psychiatric Association: Diagnostic and Statistical Manual of Mental Disorders, 4th Edition, Text Revision. Washington, DC, American Psychiatric Association, 2000

CHAPTER 36

Bulimia Nervosa

Select the single best response for each question.

36.1   A number of studies have reported the prevalence of bulimia nervosa in young women to be in the range of

A. 1%–4%.
B. 5%–10%.
C. 11%–15%.
D. 16%–20%.
E. 21%–25%.

The correct response is option A.

Several studies (Fairburn et al. 1991; Garfinkel et al. 1995; Johnson et al. 1999; Kaltiala-Heino et al. 1999; Timmerman et al. 1990; Whitaker et al. 1990) have reported bulimia nervosa prevalence rates ranging between 1% and 4%. **(p. 691)**

36.2   DSM-IV-TR (American Psychiatric Association 2000) diagnostic criteria for bulimia nervosa include all of the following *except*

A. The individual engages in recurrent episodes of binge eating.
B. The individual engages in recurrent inappropriate compensatory behavior to prevent weight gain.
C. Binge eating and inappropriate compensatory behaviors both occur, on average, at least weekly for 6 months.
D. Self-evaluation is unduly influenced by body shape and weight.
E. The disturbance does not occur exclusively during episodes of anorexia nervosa.

The correct response is option C.

Binge eating and inappropriate compensatory behaviors both occur, on average, at least twice a week for 3 months. **(p. 693)**

36.3   Compared with normal-weight individuals, persons with bulimia nervosa demonstrate elevations of which of the following neuropeptides and hormones?

A. Neuropeptide Y.
B. Cholecystokinin.
C. Leptin.
D. Cortisol.
E. None of the above.

The correct response is option A.

Neuropeptide Y and peptide YY have been shown to be elevated in patients with bulimia nervosa. Lower levels of cholecystokinin have been found in women with bulimia. Plasma leptin concentration is significantly higher in bulimic patients than in those with anorexia nervosa, but it tends to be lower than the level found in healthy control subjects. (p. 694)

36.4   In a 5-year follow-up study by Barnett (1997), risk factors demonstrated to influence the etiology of bulimia nervosa included all of the following *except*

A. Overinternalization of the value of thinness in women.
B. Inordinate dissatisfaction with body form.
C. Anxiety.
D. Depression.
E. Irrational beliefs and cognitions about thinness.

The correct response is option C.

Anxiety was not a risk factor in the etiology of bulimia nervosa in Barnett's (1997) study. (p. 695)

36.5   Which of the following antidepressants has been studied most extensively in bulimia nervosa and has been shown to be effective in its treatment?

A. Venlafaxine.
B. Mirtazapine.
C. Fluvoxamine.
D. Bupropion.
E. Fluoxetine.

The correct response is option E.

Fluoxetine is the most studied and effective antidepressant used in the treatment of bulimia nervosa. (p. 700)

References

American Psychiatric Association: Diagnostic and Statistical Manual of Mental Disorders, 4th Edition, Text Revision. Washington, DC, American Psychiatric Association, 2000

Barnett TE: Risk factors and bulimia outcomes in adolescent women: a longitudinal and retrospective analysis. Unpublished doctoral dissertation, Utah State University, 1996 [Dissertation Abstracts International 57:9-B, 5905, 1997]

Fairburn CG, Jones R, Peveler RC, et al: Three psychological treatments for bulimia nervosa: a comparative trial. Arch Gen Psychiatry 48:463–469, 1991

Garfinkel PE, Lin E, Goering P, et al: Bulimia nervosa in a Canadian community sample: prevalence and comparison of subgroups. Am J Psychiatry 152:1052–1058, 1995

Johnson C, Powers P, Dick R: Athletes and eating disorders: the National Collegiate Athletic Association Study. Int J Eat Disord 26:179–188, 1999

Kaltiala-Heino R, Rissanen A, Rimpela M, et al: Bulimia and bulimic behaviour in middle adolescence: more common than thought? Acta Psychiatr Scand 100:33–39, 1999

Timmerman MG, Wells LA, Chen S: Bulimia nervosa and associated alcohol abuse among secondary school students. J Am Acad Child Adolesc Psychiatry 29:118–122, 1990

Whitaker A, Johnson J, Sheffer D, et al: Uncommon troubles in young people: prevalence estimates of selected psychiatric disorders in a nonreferred adolescent population. Arch Gen Psychiatry 47:487–496, 1990

CHAPTER 37

Tic Disorders

Select the single best response for each question.

37.1   Which of the following statements regarding transient tic disorder is *true?*

A. Transient tics are very rare among prepubertal children.
B. Girls are more often affected than boys.
C. Transient tics run a waxing and waning course.
D. Transient tics most commonly involve the trunk and lower extremities.
E. Transient vocal tics are common.

The correct response is option C.

Transient tics run a waxing and waning course, which is often exacerbated by stress, excitement, or fatigue. Transient tics are very common in prepubertal children, with boys being more often affected than girls. Transient tics most commonly involve the face, head, neck, or arms. Transient vocal tics are much more rare. **(p. 710)**

37.2   All of the following statements regarding Tourette's syndrome are correct *except*

A. Chronic motor and phonic tic disorder was first described in 1885 by Georges Gilles de la Tourette.
B. Initial symptoms of Tourette's syndrome most frequently appear between the ages of 5 and 8 years.
C. Tic symptoms may wax and wane over time.
D. Vocal tics usually precede motor tics.
E. Children may be able to suppress tics for periods of time.

The correct response is option D.

The onset of motor tics usually precedes that of vocal tics by a year or two. **(p. 711)**

37.3   The most likely neuroanatomical substrate of Tourette's syndrome is

A. The thalamus.
B. The pituitary.
C. The prefrontal cortex.
D. The basal ganglia.
E. The amygdala.

The correct response is option D.

The basal ganglia and their connections represent the most likely neuroanatomical substrate of Tourette's syndrome. **(p. 715)**

37.4   Which of the following psychotropic agents is *least* likely to exacerbate tics?

   A. Haloperidol.
   B. L-dopa.
   C. Dextroamphetamine.
   D. Methylphenidate.
   E. Cocaine.

The correct response is option A.

Neuroleptics (e.g., haloperidol) are clinically useful in suppressing tics. Dopaminergic agonists (e.g., dextroamphetamine, methylphenidate, cocaine) frequently exacerbate tics. **(p. 716)**

37.5   Side effects of clonidine in the treatment of tic disorders include all of the following *except*

   A. Sedation.
   B. Irritability.
   C. Dry mouth.
   D. Cardiac arrhythmias.
   E. Hypertension.

The correct response is option E.

Hypertension is not a side effect of clonidine. Sedation is the primary side effect of clonidine, seen in about 10%–20% of patients. Other side effects include irritability, dry mouth, orthostatic hypotension, and, rarely, cardiac arrhythmias. **(p. 719)**

C H A P T E R 3 8

Sleep Disorders in Infancy Through Adolescence

Select the single best response for each question.

38.1   Characteristics of non–rapid eye movement (NREM) sleep include all of the following *except*

    A. Sleep spindles.
    B. K complexes.
    C. Active inhibition of muscle tone.
    D. Delta waves.
    E. Slowed and regular respiratory and heart rates.

The correct response is option C.

In NREM sleep, the active inhibition of muscle tone characteristic of the rapid eye movement (REM) state ceases, as do the REM bursts. Sleep spindles, K complexes, and delta waves define four distinct NREM sleep stages. Both respiratory and heart rate are slowed and are more regular in rhythm. **(pp. 727–728)**

38.2   In adults, sleep typically begins with which type of sleep, which occurs mostly during the first third of sleep?

    A. REM.
    B. NREM stage 1.
    C. NREM stage 2.
    D. NREM stage 3.
    E. NREM stage 4.

The correct response is option E.

In adults, sleep typically begins with NREM stage 4 sleep, and the first third of the sleep period contains most of the total night's stage 4 NREM sleep. **(p. 728)**

38.3   All of the following are classified as dyssomnias in DSM-IV-TR (American Psychiatric Association 2000) *except*

    A. Narcolepsy.
    B. Sleep terror disorder.
    C. Primary insomnia.
    D. Primary hypersomnia.
    E. Circadian rhythm sleep disorders.

The correct response is option B.

Narcolepsy, primary insomnia, primary hypersomnia, breathing-related sleep disorder, and circadian rhythm sleep disorders are classified as dyssomnias. Sleep terror disorder, nightmare disorder, and sleepwalking disorder are classified as parasomnias. **(p. 729, Table 38–1)**

38.4   Nighttime awakenings in infants have been categorized as either "signaled" or "self-soothing." Which of the following is a characteristic of self-soothing infants?

A. Self-soothers are more likely to be placed in their cribs while awake.
B. Self-soothers are more likely to use a sleep aid, such as a pacifier, to fall asleep.
C. Self-soothers may awaken for 3–5 minutes during the night but are able to fall asleep again on their own.
D. All of the above.
E. None of the above.

The correct response is option D.

Self-soothers are more likely to be placed in their cribs while awake and allowed to fall asleep on their own; signalers are placed in their cribs after they are already asleep. **(p. 731)**

38.5   Common features of NREM parasomnias include all of the following *except*

A. A predominance in males.
B. A strong positive family history.
C. Retrograde amnesia for the event on the following morning.
D. Distress upon awakening.
E. None of the above.

The correct response is option D.

NREM parasomnias are more common in children than the REM parasomnias, also known as REM sleep behavior disorders. NREM parasomnias generally occur at the end of an NREM stage 4 sleep period, just before transition to REM sleep. Common features of NREM parasomnias include a male predominance (male-to-female ratio of 6–8 to 1), a strongly positive family history, and a retrograde amnesia for the event on the following morning. Children who have parasomnias distress their families but are often not aware of their own episodes. **(p. 734)**

38.6   Characteristics of narcolepsy include all of the following *except*

A. Irresistible attacks of NREM sleep.
B. Cataplexy.
C. Hypnagogic hallucinations.
D. Sleep paralysis.
E. None of the above.

The correct response is option A.

Full-blown narcolepsy is characterized by irresistible attacks of REM sleep, cataplexy, hypnagogic hallucinations, and sleep paralysis. **(p. 737)**

Reference

American Psychiatric Association: Diagnostic and Statistical Manual of Mental Disorders, 4th Edition, Text Revision. Washington, DC, American Psychiatric Association, 2000

CHAPTER 39

Disorders of Elimination

Select the single best response for each question.

39.1 Which of the following statements regarding the clinical presentation of enuresis is *true?*

A. About 80% of patients with enuresis have primary enuresis.
B. Without treatment, the remission rate is 30%–50% per year, which decreases with age.
C. Enuresis continues into adulthood in approximately 8% of cases.
D. There is no identified increase prevalence of emotional–behavioral disorders in the enuretic population, when compared to the general population.
E. Clear association between enuresis and tic disorders has been demonstrated.

The correct response is option A.

About 80% of patients with enuresis have primary enuresis. Left untreated, the remission rate is 10%–20% per year, which gradually increases with age. Enuresis continues into adulthood in 1% of patients. The prevalence of emotional–behavioral disorders in children with enuresis is greater than in the general population. No association has been demonstrated between enuresis and tics, nail biting, temper tantrums, fire setting, or cruelty to animals. **(p. 743)**

39.2 Which of the following circumstances would be consistent with a child meeting DSM-IV-TR (American Psychiatric Association 2000) diagnostic criteria for enuresis?

A. The child must be at least 3 years of age and demonstrate repeated voiding of urine in his or her bed or clothes at least twice weekly for 3 consecutive months.
B. The child must be at least 3 years of age and demonstrate repeated voiding of urine in his or her bed or clothes at least five times weekly for 6 consecutive months.
C. The child must be at least 3 years of age and demonstrate repeated voiding of urine in his or her bed or clothes that is not due to a physiological condition.
D. The child must be at least 5 years of age and demonstrate repeated voiding of urine in his or her bed or clothes at least twice weekly for 3 consecutive months.
E. The child must be at least 5 years of age and demonstrate repeated voiding of urine in his or her bed or clothes at least five times weekly for 6 consecutive months.

The correct response is option D.

The child must be at least 5 years of age and must void urine in bed or clothes at least twice a week for at least 3 consecutive months. This behavior must not be due to the direct physiological effect of a substance (e.g., a diuretic) or a general medical condition (e.g., spina bifida). **(p. 744)**

39.3 All of the following statements regarding treatment of enuresis are correct *except*

A. Enuresis is largely a self-limited, benign disorder.
B. It is important to provide reassurance support to prevent secondary emotional effects.
C. Treatment should be preceded by a period of observation and tracking of symptoms.

D. The most effective treatment for primary enuresis is the enuresis alarm.
E. Pharmacological interventions include desmopressin (DDAVP), imipramine, and methylphenidate.

The correct response is option E.

Whereas tricyclic antidepressants, especially imipramine, and DDAVP have proved beneficial in the treatment of enuresis, methylphenidate, sedatives, and anticholinergic agents have not. **(pp. 744–745)**

39.4   Which of the following statements regarding encopresis is *true*?
A. Primary encopresis is not preceded by a period of fecal continence.
B. Secondary encopresis may account for 10%–20% of all cases.
C. Encopresis resulting from constipation and overflow incontinence is a rare form of the disorder.
D. Children with encopresis characterized by intentional depositing or smearing of feces are less likely to demonstrate defiant behaviors than are children with encopresis with overflow incontinence.
E. Most children with functional encopresis demonstrate severe behavioral problems.

The correct response is option A.

Primary encopresis is not preceded by a period of fecal continence. Secondary encopresis may account for as many as 50%–60% of all cases. Encopresis with constipation and overflow incontinence is the most common type. Children with encopresis characterized by intentional depositing or smearing of feces demonstrate more defiant behaviors than do children with encopresis with overflow incontinence. Most children with functional encopresis do not appear to have significant behavioral problems. **(p. 746)**

39.5   Which of the following statements regarding the treatment of encopresis is *true*?
A. Treatment typically includes medical interventions alone.
B. Treatment requires little evaluation because of the ease with which encopresis is diagnosed.
C. Treatment in children who retain feces should include education, disimpaction, and bowel training.
D. Treatment should not include aversive consequences for soiling accidents.
E. Biofeedback appears to be the most effective available treatment.

The correct response is option C.

The treatment principles for children who retain feces include educating the child and the parents about the problem, disimpacting the bowel, and training the child in bowel control. Medical, behavioral, and psychotherapeutic interventions should be used in the treatment of encopresis. Careful evaluation should precede any intervention. Aversive consequences for soiling accidents, such as showering and washing the soiled clothes, reinforce the child's self-monitoring. The initial promise of biofeedback therapy was not supported by subsequent studies. **(pp. 747–748)**

Reference

American Psychiatric Association: Diagnostic and Statistical Manual of Mental Disorders, 4th Edition, Text Revision. Washington, DC, American Psychiatric Association, 2000

C H A P T E R   4 0

Somatoform Disorders

Select the single best response for each question.

40.1 A useful construct, for the purpose of clinical practice, is the separation of illness into five phases. Which of the following represents the correct sequence of these phases?

A. Vulnerability to disease, adaptation or reaction to the illness, symptom onset, recurrence, chronicity of the disease state.
B. Vulnerability to disease, symptom onset, recurrence, chronicity of the disease state, adaptation or reaction to the illness.
C. Vulnerability to disease, adaptation or reaction to the illness, chronicity of the disease state, symptom onset, recurrence.
D. Adaptation or reaction to the illness, vulnerability to disease, symptom onset, recurrence, chronicity of the disease state.
E. Adaptation or reaction to the illness, vulnerability to disease, chronicity of the disease state, symptom onset, recurrence.

The correct response is option B.

The five phases of illness are vulnerability to disease, symptom onset, recurrence, chronicity of the disease state, and adaptation or reaction to the illness. **(p. 753)**

40.2 For the child psychiatrist attempting to assess the contribution of psychosocial factors to a particular patient's symptoms or illness, several key principles should be kept in mind. Which of the following is *not* one of these key principles?

A. A significant psychosomatic element is possible in every disorder.
B. A lack of satisfying findings on physical examination is adequate evidence for ascribing a psychological explanation to a specific case.
C. Even in diseases in which psychosocial factors have been widely recognized, it is possible for the psychological components to be only minimally important for a particular child's illness.
D. A lack of typical major psychopathology diagnosable in either the child or the family does not preclude the possibility that psychological factors are influencing the illness to a significant degree.
E. Psychiatric examination should identify a combination of intrapsychic and environmental factors of sufficient magnitude and likelihood to affect the course of the disorder before psychosocial intervention is undertaken.

The correct response is option B.

A lack of conclusive findings on physical or laboratory examination is not an adequate rationale for assigning a psychological explanation to a specific case. The child psychiatrist should keep in mind that a significant psychosomatic element is possible in every disorder and that even in diseases in which psychosocial factors have been widely recognized, such as asthma, diabetes, or ulcerative colitis, it is possible for the psychological components to be only minimally important for a particular child's illness. (p. 757)

40.3 Which of the following statements concerning the psychological evaluation of a child with a physical illness is *false*?

A. Especially important in the history is a chronology of the relationship between physical symptoms and emotional or stressful periods.
B. Standard psychological assessment instruments are particularly useful with children who are physically ill.
C. Having the child or parents keep a journal in which daily entries track important variables can be an asset in understanding a complicated picture.
D. Physiological measures can be helpful in the psychosomatic assessment of specific children.
E. None of the above.

The correct response is option B.

Standard psychological assessment instruments may be of limited utility with children who are physically ill, because disease-related symptoms complicate efforts to quantify psychological phenomena such as depression and anxiety. (pp. 757–758)

40.4 Which of the following would *not* be an appropriate guideline for clinicians working with families who resist psychiatric evaluation?

A. Establish a final etiological diagnosis.
B. Concentrate on the psychosocial history, common sources of stress, family psychiatric history, and emotional consequences of the dysfunction.
C. Suggest focusing on the dysfunction rather than on a diagnosis.
D. Advocate patience, with the hope that time will foster a sufficient relationship.
E. Suggest an "if–then" approach, encouraging the family to agree in advance to accept a referral if the last round of diagnostic test results are negative.

The correct response is option A.

Clinicians should avoid making a final etiological diagnosis; instead, they should suggest to the family that because both the physical and the psychological components of the child's illness require further exploration, the evaluation should focus on dysfunction rather than diagnosis. (pp. 758–759)

40.5 Which of the following would *not* be an appropriate guideline for a clinician initiating therapy with a chronically ill child and his or her family?

A. The therapist must respect the reality of the medical situation.
B. The therapist must confront the family's somatic disposition early in therapy, encouraging them to think and speak in psychological, not somatic, terms.
C. The therapist must respect the patient's creativity in discovering coping solutions.
D. The therapist must bear in mind that the standards used for judging mental health, defenses, and developmental progression in physically healthy children often do not apply or are only partially relevant to children with chronic illness.
E. The therapist must refrain from underestimating or minimizing the stressors associated with having a chronic or potentially fatal illness.

The correct response is option B.

The therapist must respect the patient's and family's need for somatic language and symptoms (i.e., their need to think and speak in terms of physical illness, medical problems, and bodily dysfunction). The therapist must also respect the reality of the medical situation and the patient's creativity in discovering coping solutions. **(p. 759)**

CHAPTER 41

Adjustment and Reactive Disorders

Select the single best response for each question.

41.1 The diagnosis of adjustment disorder in children and adolescents

A. Has a focus similar to that in other psychiatric disorders, emphasizing observable symptoms and internalized experiences as primary components of the condition.

B. Elevates the importance of families and outside systems because of its emphasis on psychosocial stressors.

C. Requires that symptoms develop within 6 months of the onset of the stressors.

D. Requires that the presenting symptoms be similar to what would be expected for any child exposed to the stressor in question.

E. Is warranted when symptoms continue for years after the termination of the stressor.

The correct response is option B.

The diagnosis of adjustment disorder elevates the importance of involving families and outside systems in treatment, because its focus is on the connection between stressors and psychological distress. DSM-IV-TR (American Psychiatric Association 2000) criteria require that symptoms occur within 3 months of the onset of the stressor and that symptoms be beyond what would be expected in other children meeting a similar stressor. In addition, symptoms should resolve within 6 months of the termination of the stressor or its consequences. **(p. 767)**

41.2 Which of the following statements regarding cultural syndromes and issues affecting child and adolescent patients is *true?*

A. Cultural syndromes are considered pathological conditions.

B. Cultural syndromes may be best understood by obtaining collateral information from family members or others knowledgeable about the individual's culture.

C. Changes in functioning that do not exceed the bounds of culturally sanctioned phenomena are likely to have long-term negative sequelae.

D. In a study by Bird et al. (1989), the authors reported the culturally specific finding that Puerto Rican children in single-parent families had higher rates of childhood psychopathology than did U.S. mainland children in single-parent families.

E. Bird et al. (1989) suggested that the prominent role played by extended families in the U.S. likely was protective for these children.

The correct response is option B.

Collateral information from family members or other members of the individual's culture of origin may be necessary to distinguish pathological symptoms from cultural phenomena. Cultural syndromes are not considered to be pathological disorders. Changes in functioning that do not exceed the bounds of culturally sanctioned phenomena are considered "normal" and would not be expected to have negative long-term sequelae. In the Bird et al. (1989) study, single parenthood was not associated with the psychopathology variables in Puerto Rican children. It was believed that the prominent role of the extended family in Puerto Rico might serve as a protective factor in single-parent families, shielding the child from the development of symptoms. **(p. 768)**

41.3   All of the following factors can likely amplify the impact of an identifiable stressor on a child *except*

    A. Cognitive immaturity.
    B. Preexisting low self-esteem.
    C. More primitive defense mechanisms.
    D. More accurate understanding of cause-and-effect relationships.
    E. Treatment side effects.

The correct response is option D.

Children are more likely than adults to link unrelated events as cause-and-effect phenomena. **(p. 769)**

41.4   In Kovacs et al.'s (1994) controlled prospective study of children with adjustment disorder, which of the following findings was reported?

    A. More than half of the study group children reported a history of suicidal ideation after the onset of the stressor.
    B. More than half of the study population had suffered the death of a parent.
    C. The median time to recovery after symptom onset was 3 months.
    D. Close to 100% recovery was reported in the study population within 12 months.
    E. The study group evidenced significantly more long-term sequelae compared with the control group.

The correct response is option A.

In the study of Kovacs et al. (1994), more than half (58%) of the children indicated a history of suicidal ideation at some point after onset of the stressor. Only 7% of the children studied had suffered the death of a parent or grandparent. The median time to recovery was 7 months, and close to 100% of the study population had resolution of symptoms within 2 years. Compared with the control group, there was no evidence of long-term sequelae over an 8-year follow-up assessment. **(p. 769)**

41.5   In Kovacs et al.'s (1995) study of children hospitalized for acute-onset diabetes, all of the following findings were reported *except*

    A. Seventy-three percent of adjustment disorder diagnoses were made during the first month after the diabetes diagnosis.
    B. The first month posthospitalization was the period of greatest psychological vulnerability.
    C. Greater vulnerability during the first month postdiagnosis may be related to physiological factors.
    D. Short-term psychiatric outcomes for the study population were poor.
    E. The presence of adjustment disorder was a risk factor for developing other psychiatric illnesses within the next 5 years.

The correct response is option D.

The short-term psychiatric outcomes for the children in this study were good (Kovacs et al. 1995). All of the children eventually recovered from the adjustment disorder, with the average time to recovery being 3 months. **(p. 771)**

References

American Psychiatric Association: Diagnostic and Statistical Manual of Mental Disorders, 4th Edition, Text Revision. Washington, DC, American Psychiatric Association, 2000

Bird HR, Gould MS, Yager T, et al: Risk factors for maladjustment in Puerto Rican children. J Am Acad Child Adolesc Psychiatry 28:847–850, 1989

Kovacs M, Gatsonis C, Pollock M, et al: A controlled prospective study of DSM-III adjustment disorder in childhood: short-term prognosis and long-term predictive validity. Arch Gen Psychiatry 51:535–541, 1994

Kovacs M, Ho V, Pollock MH: Criterion and predictive validity of the diagnosis of adjustment disorder: a prospective study of youths with new-onset insulin-dependent diabetes mellitus. Am J Psychiatry 152:523–528, 1995

C H A P T E R 4 2

Personality Disorders

Select the single best response for each question.

42.1 In DSM-IV-TR (American Psychiatric Association 2000), personality disorder categories may be applied to children and adolescents if which of the following criteria is satisfied?

A. The maladaptive personality traits appear to be pervasive and persistent.
B. The maladaptive personality traits appeared before age 12 years.
C. The maladaptive personality traits have been present for at least 6 months.
D. The maladaptive traits appeared before age 7 years.
E. None of the above.

The correct response is option A.

DSM-IV-TR indicates that personality disorder categories may be applied to children or adolescents in the relatively unusual instance in which the individual's particular maladaptive personality traits appear to be pervasive and persistent, or in individuals younger than 18 years whose maladaptive features have been present for at least 1 year. **(p. 775)**

42.2 The New York Longitudinal Study (Thomas and Chess 1977) showed that between the ages of 3 months and 2 years, the *least* stable personality characteristic was

A. Mood.
B. Activity level.
C. Adaptability.
D. Approach behavior.
E. Intensity.

The correct response is option B.

Activity level and distractibility were the least stable personality traits during this period, whereas mood, adaptability, approach behavior, and intensity were the most stable. **(p. 777)**

42.3 In DSM-IV-TR, personality disorders are grouped into clusters. Into which cluster do avoidant, dependent, and obsessive-compulsive personality disorders fall?

A. Cluster A.
B. Cluster B.
C. Cluster C.
D. Cluster D.
E. None of the above.

The correct response is option C.

Avoidant, dependent, and obsessive-compulsive categories are grouped in Cluster C. Cluster A includes paranoid, schizoid, and schizotypal personality disorders, whereas Cluster B includes the antisocial, borderline, histrionic, and narcissistic categories. **(p. 778)**

42.4   Diagnostic criteria for histrionic personality disorder include all of the following *except*

   A. Is uncomfortable in situations in which he or she is not the center of attention.
   B. Displays rapidly shifting and shallow expression of emotions.
   C. Shows self-dramatization.
   D. Experiences chronic feelings of emptiness.
   E. Is suggestible.

   The correct response is option D.

   Chronic feelings of emptiness are not included in the diagnostic criteria for histrionic personality disorder but are characteristic of another cluster B category, borderline personality disorder. **(pp. 780–781)**

42.5   Children with borderline personality disorder commonly

   A. Report kinesthetic and tactile hallucinations.
   B. Play in an age-appropriate manner.
   C. Exhibit empathy for others.
   D. Have surprisingly good relationships with peers.
   E. Play in a compulsive fashion, without evidence of enjoyment.

   The correct response is option E.

   Children with borderline personality disorder do not play in an age-appropriate manner. Their play is compulsive, with little evidence of enjoyment or of the capacity to resolve conflict. **(p. 782)**

References

American Psychiatric Association: Diagnostic and Statistical Manual of Mental Disorders, 4th Edition, Text Revision. Washington, DC, American Psychiatric Association, 2000

Thomas A, Chess S: Temperament and Development. New York, Brunner/Mazel, 1977

CHAPTER 43

Substance Abuse Disorders

Select the single best response for each question.

43.1 Which of the following has been reported to be a problem in applying DSM-IV-TR (American Psychiatric Association 2000) criteria to adolescents?

A. Withdrawal and drug-related medical problems are common.
B. One abuse symptom yields a diagnosis.
C. Abuse symptoms frequently precede dependence symptoms.
D. Two dependence symptoms with no abuse symptoms yields a diagnosis.
E. None of the above.

The correct response is option B.

In the DSM-IV-TR criteria, one abuse symptom yields a diagnosis. In adolescents, however, abuse symptoms often do not precede dependence symptoms. Under the DSM-IV-TR criteria, an adolescent with two dependence symptoms but no abuse symptoms would not qualify for a diagnosis, although such an individual would need therapeutic intervention. Withdrawal and drug-related medical problems are rare, not common, in youth. **(p. 796)**

43.2 In the 2001 Monitoring the Future Survey (Johnston et al. 2001), epidemiological findings concerning substance abuse in high school seniors included all of the following *except*

A. Marijuana use by about 37%.
B. Cigarette smoking during the past month by 29.5%.
C. MDMA (3,4-methylenedioxymethamphetamine; "ecstasy") use by 9.2%.
D. Anabolic steroid use by 12.4%.
E. Alcohol use by about 73%.

The correct response is option D.

In 2001, only 2.4% of high school seniors reported the use of anabolic steroids (Johnston et al. 2001). **(pp. 796–797)**

43.3 The well-known CAGE screening questions developed for adults are not useful for adolescents. The CRAFFT, a screening instrument developed for adolescents, includes all of the following questions *except*

A. "Have you ever ridden in a Car driven by someone (including yourself) who was high or had been using alcohol or drugs?"
B. "Do you ever use alcohol/drugs to Relax, feel better about yourself, or fit in?"
C. "Do you get Angry when you are told that you have a problem?"
D. "Do you ever Forget things you did while using alcohol/drugs?"
E. "Have you ever gotten into Trouble while you were using alcohol/drugs?"

The correct response is option C.

The CRAFFT screen includes all of the questions above except for that in option C. The correct question corresponding to the letter *A* in *CRAFFT* is "Do you ever use alcohol/drugs while you are by yourself or Alone?" The CRAFFT also includes a second *F* question—"Do your Family or Friends ever tell you that you should cut down on your drinking or drug use?" Two or more "yes" answers suggest serious problems with substances and indicate the need for further evaluation (Knight et al. 1999). **(p. 799)**

43.4   Risk factors for the development of substance abuse disorders include all of the following *except*

A. Economic and social advantage.
B. School failure.
C. Friends who use drugs.
D. Psychiatric comorbidity.
E. History of parental divorce.

The correct response is option A.

Economic and social *deprivation*, rather than advantage, is a risk factor for substance abuse. **(p. 800, Table 43–3)**

43.5   A common comorbid diagnosis in male adolescents with substance abuse is

A. Conduct disorder.
B. Attention-deficit/hyperactivity disorder.
C. Avoidant personality disorder.
D. Oppositional defiant disorder.
E. None of the above.

The correct response is option A.

Conduct disorder and antisocial personality disorder are the most common comorbid diagnoses with substance abuse, particularly in males. **(p. 808)**

References

American Psychiatric Association: Diagnostic and Statistical Manual of Mental Disorders, 4th Edition, Text Revision. Washington, DC, American Psychiatric Association, 2000

Johnston LD, O'Malley PM, Bachman JG: National Survey Results on Drug Use From the Monitoring the Future Study, 1975–2000, Vol 1: Secondary School Students (NIH Publ No 01-4924). Rockville, MD, National Institute on Drug Abuse, 2001

Knight JR, Shrier LA, Bravender TD, et al: A new brief screen for adolescent substance abuse. Arch Pediatr Adolesc Med 153:591–596, 1999

C H A P T E R 4 4

Gender Identity and Psychosexual Disorders

Select the single best response for each question.

44.1   Which of the following statements concerning gender identity is *false*?

   A. Gender identity typically appears in its nascent form between 2 and 3 years of age.
   B. Children 2–3 years of age are able to categorize people by sex on the basis of phenotypic social cues, such as clothing or hairstyle.
   C. *Gender identity* refers to a person's behavioral adoption of cultural markers of masculinity and femininity.
   D. The ability to categorize others by sex likely precedes the ability to self-categorize oneself as a boy or girl.
   E. None of the above.

The correct response is option C.

Gender identity refers to a person's basic sense of self as male or female. It includes both the awareness that one is male or female and an affective appraisal of such knowledge. **(p. 813)**

44.2   In children, according to DSM-IV-TR (American Psychiatric Association 2000), gender identity disorder is manifested by which of the following?

   A. A repeatedly stated desire to be, or insistence that he or she is, the other sex.
   B. Strong and persistent preferences for cross-sex roles in make-believe play.
   C. An intense desire to participate in the stereotypical games and pastimes of the other sex.
   D. A strong preference for playmates of the other sex.
   E. All of the above.

The correct response is option E.

All of the above are manifested in children with gender identity disorder. **(p. 814, Table 44–1)**

44.3   The age at onset of cross-gender behavior in gender identity disorder is typically

   A. Before the age of 5 years.
   B. Between the ages of 6 and 10 years.
   C. Between the ages of 12 and 15 years.
   D. Between the ages of 16 and 19 years.
   E. None of the above.

The correct response is option A.

Green (1976) reported that the age at onset of cross-gender behaviors in gender identity disorder is typically during the preschool years. Many experienced clinicians have observed that repetitive, intense cross-gender behaviors appear even before a child's second birthday. **(p. 818)**

44.4 Which of the following statements concerning biophysical markers in children with gender identity disorder is *true*?

A. Standard endocrine assessments frequently detect abnormalities.
B. Abnormal XY karyotypes have been reported in boys.
C. Feminine boys are shorter and weigh less than nonfeminine boys at the time of assessment.
D. All of the above.
E. None of the above.

The correct response is option E.

Because sex hormone levels are so low during childhood, it is unlikely that a standard endocrine assessment would detect abnormalities. Abnormal XY karyotypes have not been found in boys with gender identity disorder. Feminine boys do not differ from nonfeminine boys in height and weight at the time of assessment. **(p. 819)**

44.5 Scholars who have reworked the original Kinsey report concerning the prevalence of homosexuality in men (Kinsey et al. 1948) estimate rates in the range of

A. 1%–2%.
B. 2%–6%.
C. 6%–10%.
D. 10%–12%.
E. None of the above.

The correct response is option B.

Scholars who have reworked the Kinsey data have found much lower prevalence rates than the 10% reported by Kinsey et al. (1948). Current prevalence estimates for homosexuality are 2%–6% for men and about 2% for women (Diamond 1993; Rogers and Turner 1991). **(p. 821)**

References

American Psychiatric Association: Diagnostic and Statistical Manual of Mental Disorders, 4th Edition, Text Revision. Washington, DC, American Psychiatric Association, 2000

Diamond M: Homosexuality and bisexuality in different populations. Arch Sex Behav 22:291–310, 1993

Green R: One hundred ten feminine and masculine boys: behavioral contrasts and demographic similarities. Arch Sex Behav 5:425–446, 1976

Kinsey AC, Pomeroy WB, Martin CE: Sexual Behavior in the Human Male. Philadelphia, PA, WB Saunders, 1948

Rogers SM, Turner CF: Male–male sexual contact in the USA: findings from five sample surveys, 1970–1990. J Sex Res 28:491–519, 1991

CHAPTER 45

Physical Abuse of Children

Select the single best response for each question.

45.1   Which of the following statements concerning the epidemiology of physical abuse of children is *false?*

A.   Younger children (less than 3 years of age) have the greatest risk of fatal maltreatment.
B.   Homicides occurring during the first week of life are almost exclusively perpetrated by mothers.
C.   Fathers are more likely to fatally injure their children ages 1 week to 13 years.
D.   Fathers committed the majority of parent-perpetrated homicides of children 13–19 years of age.
E.   None of the above.

The correct response is option C.

Mothers and fathers are equally likely to fatally injure their children ages 1 week to 13 years. **(p. 837)**

45.2   Risk factors that may predict recurrence of abuse in children include which of the following?

A.   Young age of the child.
B.   Number of previous referrals to child protective services.
C.   History of childhood abuse in the caretaker.
D.   Prematurity, mental retardation, or physical handicaps in the child.
E.   All of the above.

The correct response is option E.

In addition to all of the above factors, a history of low birth weight or cognitive or neuropsychiatric deficits make children more vulnerable to maltreatment. **(p. 838)**

45.3   Indicators suggesting possible physical abuse in a child who presents with an injury include all of the following *except*

A.   Observation of an inappropriate history for the injury.
B.   A reasonable explanation for the injury.
C.   An excessive or inadequate level of concern in the parent.
D.   Delay in seeking medical attention.
E.   A contradictory, changing, or vague history of the injury.

The correct response is option B.

A reasonable explanation for the injury is not present. In addition, a parent who blames an injury on a sibling or claims that it was self-inflicted, or a parent with unrealistic or premature expectations of the child, could also be suggestive of abuse. **(p. 839)**

45.4   Which of the following characteristics in children should increase a clinician's suspicion of possible physical abuse?

A. A child who is afraid to leave home.
B. A child who craves physical contact.
C. A child with excessive needs for being comforted.
D. A child who is on the alert for danger.
E. All of the above.

The correct response is option D.

Indicative characteristics include a child who is unusually fearful, docile, distrustful, or guarded; a child with no expectation of being comforted; a child who is wary of physical contact; a child who is on the alert for danger; a child who attempts to meet parents' needs by role reversal; and a child who is afraid to go home. **(pp. 839–840)**

45.5   Physical findings in an injured child suggestive of physical abuse include which of the following?

A. Bruises or lacerations in the shape of an object.
B. Posterior rib fractures.
C. Anogenital lacerations.
D. Twisting injuries of the ear lobe.
E. All of the above.

The correct response is option E.

Other suggestive findings include burns, head injuries, ruptured tympanic membranes, multiple fractures in different stages of healing, abdominal injuries, and chest injuries. **(p. 840)**

CHAPTER 46

Sexual Abuse of Children

Select the single best response for each question.

46.1   Which of the following statements concerning sexual abuse of boys is *false?*

A. Perpetrators of abuse against boys are most likely to be related to the victim.
B. Boys are less likely than girls to disclose abuse.
C. Surveys indicate that as many as 18% of males older than 18 years report having been victims of childhood sexual abuse.
D. Perpetrators of abuse against boys are most likely to be male.
E. Sexual abuse of boys may be significantly underreported and untreated.

The correct response is option A.

Perpetrators of abuse against boys are most likely to be male and unrelated to the victim. **(p. 855)**

46.2   In comparison with the general population, persons who perpetrate sexual abuse

A. Are more frequently from lower socioeconomic classes.
B. Are less likely to have been raised in families with a history of domestic violence.
C. Are more likely to have been abused as children.
D. Are less likely to be practicing a religion.
E. Are more often of minority race/ethnicity.

The correct response is option C.

It is commonly believed that abusers often were themselves abused as children. Sexual abuse is prevalent in all socioeconomic classes, and abusers have a racial, religious, and ethnic profile similar to that of the general population. **(p. 855)**

46.3   Perpetrators of sexual abuse

A. Are often children and adolescents.
B. Are gender specific regarding their choice of victims.
C. Often associate themselves with events or activities in which they have access to children.
D. May seek to "groom" victims with gifts or money.
E. All of the above.

The correct response is option E.

Perpetrators may associate with youth group activities, schools, recreational facilities, or locations near playgrounds. They may seek to "groom" potential victims by offering gifts or money in order to gain their trust. Perpetrators are most often male and most often select female victims. They are usually gender specific in their choice of victims; those who select both male and female victims may have more severe psychopathology. Approximately 30%–50% of assaults are perpetrated by children and adolescents younger than 18 years of age. **(p. 856)**

46.4   Psychiatric disorders often found in sexually abused children include all of the following *except*

   A. Depression.
   B. Bipolar disorder.
   C. Anxiety disorders.
   D. Schizophrenia.
   E. Eating disorders.

   The correct response is option D.

   Schizophrenia is not normally found in sexually abused children. In addition to the categories listed above, disruptive behavior disorders with prominent symptoms of aggression, hyperactivity, and motor restlessness, and posttraumatic stress disorder, are also prominent. **(pp. 858–859)**

46.5   Key points to consider when conducting a forensic evaluation of a child for suspected sexual abuse include all of the following *except*

   A. A stepwise interview approach, starting with nonabuse topics and progressing to abuse topics, works best.
   B. Psychological testing and screening checklists may provide definitive evidence of abuse.
   C. A gentle, nonthreatening demeanor that avoids retraumatization is essential.
   D. Biased or leading questions should be avoided.
   E. Specialized techniques, such as the use of drawings or anatomical dolls, may be useful for younger children but are not essential.

   The correct response is option B.

   Psychologist testing and screening checklists may be useful for treatment purposes but do not provide definitive evidence of sexual abuse. **(p. 861)**

CHAPTER 47

HIV and AIDS:
Global and United States
Perspectives

Select the single best response for each question.

47.1   All of the following statistics concerning human immunodeficiency virus (HIV)/acquired
       immunodeficiency syndrome (AIDS) worldwide in 2002 are correct *except*

   A. 3.2 million children younger than 15 years of age were living with HIV/AIDS.
   B. 800,000 children became newly infected with HIV.
   C. Less than 100,000 children younger than 15 years of age died of AIDS.
   D. 19.2 million women were infected with HIV/AIDS.
   E. 1.2 million women died of AIDS.

   The correct response is option C.

   During 2002, a total of 3.1 million people died of AIDS, including 610,000 children younger than 15
   years of age (Joint United Nations Programme on HIV/AIDS 2002). AIDS has become the fourth-
   largest cause of death worldwide. In the developing world, the majority of new infections occur in
   young women of childbearing age and in young children, who are especially vulnerable. **(p. 869)**

47.2   As of June 2001, the most common exposure group for U.S. children younger than 13 years of age
       with AIDS was

   A. Children born to mothers who are injection drug users or sexual partners of HIV-infected males.
   B. Children with hemophilia or coagulation disorder.
   C. Recipients of transfusion, blood components, or tissue.
   D. Undetermined.
   E. None of the above.

   The correct response is option A.

   The vast majority (91%) of AIDS patients younger than age 13 years were born to injection drug users
   or partners of males infected with HIV (Centers for Disease Control and Prevention 2001). **(p. 873)**

47.3   Which of the following is the preferred method for diagnosing HIV in infancy?
   A. HIV RNA assay in plasma.
   B. HIV culture.
   C. DNA polymerase chain reaction (PCR) assay.
   D. Presence of maternal antibodies.
   E. Enzyme-linked immunosorbent assay (ELISA).

The correct response is option C.

The DNA PCR assay is the preferred method for diagnosing HIV in infancy. **(p. 875)**

47.4 As of June 2001, the *least* common exposure route for U.S. adolescents between the ages of 13 and 19 years with AIDS was

A. High-risk sexual contact.
B. Injection drug use.
C. Blood transfusion or coagulation disorder.
D. Undetermined.
E. None of the above.

The correct response is option C.

Adolescents are least likely (4% in males, 1% in females) to contract AIDS from blood transfusions or other treatments for coagulation disorders (Centers for Disease Control and Prevention 2001). **(pp. 877–878)**

47.5 According to guidelines of the American Academy of Child and Adolescent Psychiatry (1995), HIV-infected adolescents who require inpatient psychiatric or substance abuse treatment

A. Should be denied admission.
B. Should be segregated from other patients.
C. Should be assigned to individual rooms.
D. Should be treated with universal precautionary measures, unlike HIV-negative patients.
E. None of the above.

The correct response is option E.

HIV infection should not be a reason for denying admission. *All* patients should be treated with universal precautions; hence, HIV-infected adolescents do not need to be segregated (American Academy of Child and Adolescent Psychiatry 1995). **(p. 881)**

References

American Academy of Child and Adolescent Psychiatry: Policy statement: HIV and treatment issues in children and adolescents. Washington, DC, HIV Issues Committee, American Academy of Child and Adolescent Psychiatry, 1995

Centers for Disease Control and Prevention: HIV/AIDS Surveillance Report: U.S. HIV and AIDS Cases Reported Through June 2001, Vol 13, No 1. Atlanta, GA, Centers for Disease Control and Prevention, 2001

Joint United Nations Programme on HIV/AIDS: AIDS Epidemic Update: December 2001. Geneva, Joint United Nations Programme on HIV/AIDS and World Health Organization, 2002

C H A P T E R   4 8

Suicide and Suicidality

Select the single best response for each question.

48.1   Self-mutilation

   A. Is defined as superficial cutting of the arms, legs, and other body areas.
   B. Is rarely associated with stress.
   C. Always involves a clear intention to kill oneself.
   D. Is never associated with suicidal intent.
   E. Is rarely associated with dissociative phenomena.

The correct response is option A.

Self-mutilation involves superficial cutting of the arms, legs, and other body areas and is often associated with stress, dissociative phenomena, and anger. Although often associated with suicidal intent, self-mutilation is not in itself considered to be a suicidal act. **(p. 892)**

48.2   Which of the following statements concerning epidemiological findings in youth suicide is *false?*

   A. Suicide among black youth has increased more rapidly than that among white youth.
   B. Increased rates of youth suicide are associated with greater availability of firearms.
   C. Male youths are more likely to attempt suicide than are females.
   D. Approximately 1% of preadolescents in the general population report having made a suicide attempt.
   E. None of the above.

The correct response is option C.

According to the Youth Risk Behavior Surveillance System 1999 survey (Kann et al. 2000), female adolescents were more likely to have attempted suicide than were males (10.9% vs. 5.7%).
(pp. 894–895)

48.3   Which of the following childhood environmental stressors has been identified as a suicide risk factor?

   A. Adolescent unemployment.
   B. Family history of suicidal behavior.
   C. Poor communication with the mother or the father.
   D. Adolescent suspension from school.
   E. All of the above.

The correct response is option E.

All of the above stressors have been identified as suicide risk factors (Gould et al. 1996). Other stressors include father's problem with police, mother's history of mood disorder, lack of an intact family, and loss. **(p. 893)**

48.4   A "psychological autopsy" study of 67 adolescent suicide victims found greatly elevated risks for suicide associated with certain psychiatric disorders (Brent et al. 1993). Which of the following disorders imparted the greatest increase in risk?

   A. Attention-deficit/hyperactivity disorder.
   B. Alcohol abuse.
   C. Schizophrenia.
   D. Major depression.
   E. Conduct disorder.

The correct response is option D.

Major depression imparted the highest increase for suicide, followed by drug abuse, alcohol abuse, and conduct disorder (Brent et al. 1993). **(p. 893)**

48.5   Research studies examining treatment targeted toward prevention of child and adolescent suicide have reported which of the following findings?

   A. Unlike the case in adults, depression is not a key risk factor for suicide in children and adolescents.
   B. Utilization of mental health treatment among depressed youths is high, approaching 75%.
   C. Presence or absence of health insurance coverage has little to do with whether children receive antidepressant treatment.
   D. Family functioning typically has little association with suicidal behavior in youths.
   E. Children and adolescents who attempt suicide are often first evaluated in emergency departments.

The correct response is option E.

Children and adolescents who attempt suicide are frequently first evaluated in emergency services. Although depression is a key risk factor in youth suicide and suicide attempts (Flisher 1999), utilization of mental health treatment among depressed youths is not common. In one study (Wu et al. 2001), 36% of depressed and dysthymic youth never received professional care, and of those who were treated, only 31% were treated with antidepressants. Factors associated with receipt of antidepressant treatment included mother's level of education, whether the children had health insurance, and whether the children had suicidal or other severe symptoms. Suicidal behavior has been identified as being associated with family dysfunction; however, few empirical studies have evaluated the effects of family intervention on suicidal behavior among children and adolescents. **(p. 899)**

References

Brent DA, Perper JA, Moritz G, et al: Psychiatric risk factors for adolescent suicide: a case-control study. J Am Acad Child Adolesc Psychiatry 32:521–529, 1993

Gould MS, Fisher P, Parides M, et al: Psychosocial risk factors of child and adolescent completed suicide. Arch Gen Psychiatry 53:1155–1162, 1996

Kann L, Kinchen SA, Williams BI, et al: Youth Risk Behavior Surveillance—United States, 1999. J Sch Health 70:271–285, 2000

C H A P T E R   4 9

Forensic Psychiatry

Select the single best response for each question.

49.1   The White House Conference on Children, convened in 1970 (U.S. Government Printing Office 1971), asserted all of the following specific rights as central to a child's well-being *except*

A. The right to be born and to be healthy and wanted throughout childhood.
B. The right to mental health care, regardless of socioeconomic status.
C. The right to be educated to the limits of one's capability.
D. The right to grow up nurtured by affectionate parents.
E. The right to have societal mechanisms to enforce the foregoing rights.

The correct response is option B.

Mental health care was not deemed a specific right central to a child's well-being. **(p. 904)**

49.2   Which of the following standards of proof is required in juvenile court and delinquency proceedings?

A. Reasonable degree of certainty.
B. Clear and convincing evidence.
C. Beyond a reasonable doubt.
D. Preponderance of the evidence.
E. More likely than not.

The correct response is option C.

The highest standard of proof—beyond a reasonable doubt—is required by law in criminal cases, including juvenile court and delinquency proceedings. **(p. 905)**

49.3   Special ethical dimensions that distinguish the care and treatment of children include which of the following?

A. The child is a minor, and parental involvement is necessary to some degree.
B. The child's developmental maturation expands the capacity for understanding and judgment and responsibility for behavior.
C. The child is involved with school and perhaps other social agencies and institutions that require exchange of information and collaboration in the care and treatment efforts.
D. All of the above.
E. None of the above.

The correct response is option D.

All three of the dimensions listed above must be considered in the care and treatment of children (Sondheimer and Martucci 1992). **(p. 908)**

49.4 Which of the following is *not* an element of informed consent?

   A. The clinician must inform the patient of the nature of the condition and the recommended treatment, including benefits and risks.
   B. The clinician must adhere to the professional practice standard prevailing at the time in the community.
   C. The patient's choice must be voluntary.
   D. The patient must have the capacity to consent.
   E. The clinician should inform the patient of alternatives to the recommended treatment, including their risks and benefits.

The correct response is option B.

Informed consent does not include a statement requiring the clinician to adhere to the professional practice standard prevailing at the time in the community. **(p. 911)**

49.5 The essential elements of professional malpractice include all of the following *except*

   A. A duty of care was owed to the patient by the physician.
   B. The proper diagnosis was not made.
   C. The patient experienced actual damage due to the breach of duty.
   D. The duty of care was breached.
   E. The dereliction was the direct cause of the damages.

The correct response is option B.

Misdiagnosis is not an element of professional negligence or malpractice. The essential elements are sometimes referred to as "the four *D*'s of negligence": **D**uty, **D**ereliction, **D**amages, and **D**irect causation (options A, D, C, and E above, respectively). **(p. 912)**

49.6 The current guiding principle in deciding child custody disputes is

   A. The wishes of the parent.
   B. The mental and physical health of the parents.
   C. The interactions of the child with those who may significantly affect his or her best interests.
   D. The wishes of the child.
   E. The best interests of the child.

The correct response is option E.

The legal doctrine of the best interests of the child is the guiding principle in deciding child custody disputes (Nurcombe and Partlett 1994). Other relevant factors that may be considered are the wishes of the child and parents; interactions of the child with those who affect his or her care; the child's adjustment to home, school, or community; and the mental and physical health of all individuals involved. **(p. 913)**

References

Nurcombe B, Partlett DF: Child Mental Health and the Law. New York, Free Press, 1994

Sondheimer A, Martucci LC: An approach to teaching ethics in child and adolescent psychiatry. J Am Acad Child Adolesc Psychiatry 31:415–422, 1992

U.S. Government Printing Office: Report to the President: White House Conference on Children. Washington, DC, U.S. Government Printing Office, 1971

CHAPTER 50

Psychopharmacology

Select the single best response for each question.

50.1 Commonly reported and well-substantiated side effects of stimulant medications include all of the following *except*

A. Appetite suppression.
B. Sleep disturbance.
C. Mild increases in pulse and blood pressure.
D. Stunting of growth in height.
E. Weight loss.

The correct response is option D.

Stimulants are known to routinely produce anorexia and weight loss, but their effect on growth in height is much less certain. **(pp. 934–935)**

50.2 A number of studies have evaluated the short- and long-term effects of therapeutic doses of tricyclic antidepressants (TCAs) on the cardiovascular system in children. Which of the following statements is *incorrect?*

A. TCAs are generally well tolerated.
B. TCAs may produce electrocardiographic abnormalities at doses between 1 and 2 mg/kg.
C. Patients should be carefully monitored at higher TCA doses (greater than 3.5 mg/kg).
D. Before initiating TCAs, a baseline electrocardiogram is recommended.
E. None of the above.

The correct response is option B.

TCAs are generally well tolerated, with only minor electrocardiographic changes associated with daily oral doses as high as 5.0 mg/kg. TCA-induced electrocardiographic abnormalities (conduction defects) have been consistently reported in children receiving doses higher than 3.5 mg/kg. **(p. 938)**

50.3 Some compounds metabolized by the cytochrome P450 enzyme 3A4 have been associated with QT prolongations when combined with drugs that inhibit 3A4. Antidepressants that affect 3A4 activity include all of the following *except*

A. Fluvoxamine.
B. Venlafaxine.
C. Nefazodone.
D. Fluoxetine.
E. Sertraline.

The correct response is option B.

Venlafaxine, citalopram, and mirtazapine minimally inhibit P450 enzymes. **(pp. 939–940)**

50.4 Novel atypical antipsychotic medications exert their therapeutic effects through antagonism of which of the following receptors?

A. Dopaminergic (D_1).
B. Histaminic (H_1).
C. Serotonergic (5-HT_2).
D. Alpha$_1$-adrenergic.
E. None of the above.

The correct response is option C.

Novel atypical antipsychotic medications, such as risperidone, olanzapine, and quetiapine, combine dopaminergic (D_2) and serotonergic (5-HT_2) antagonist properties and are associated with a lower incidence of acute extrapyramidal adverse effects and possibly a lower risk of tardive dyskinesia. **(p. 940)**

50.5 Oxcarbazepine is chemically similar to carbamazepine with some important differences, which include all of the following *except*

A. Laboratory monitoring is still required with oxcarbazepine.
B. Oxcarbazepine has little interaction with the cytochrome P450 system.
C. Oxcarbazepine lacks the hepatic liability of carbamazepine.
D. Oxcarbazepine does not induce its own metabolism.
E. Oxcarbazepine lacks the hematological liability of carbamazepine.

The correct response is option A.

Laboratory monitoring is *not* required, because oxcarbazepine does not share the hepatic and hematological liability of carbamazepine. **(p. 945)**

50.6 In child psychiatry, clonidine is commonly used in the treatment of all of the following *except*

A. Attention-deficit/hyperactivity disorder (ADHD).
B. Tourette's disorder.
C. Aggression.
D. Sleep disturbance in ADHD children.
E. Major depressive disorder.

The correct response is option E.

Clonidine is not used in the treatment of major depressive disorder. **(p. 947)**

50.7 Side effects associated with the use of atomoxetine in children include which of the following?

A. Increased appetite.
B. Cardiac conduction delays.
C. Insomnia.
D. Increase in pulse and diastolic blood pressure.
E. Abuse.

The correct response is option D.

In children, possible side effects of atomoxetine include mild increases in pulse and blood pressure and mild decreases in appetite. Atomoxetine does not cause insomnia or cardiac conduction or repolarization delays. In addition, atomoxetine is not abusable. **(p. 948, Table 50–7)**

C H A P T E R   5 1

Psychoanalysis and Psychodynamic Therapy

Select the single best response for each question.

51.1   Melanie Klein's technique of child psychoanalysis is based on which of the following fundamental principles?

A. Verbalization and clarification of the preconscious material.
B. Suggestions and educational efforts.
C. Play as the child's mode of free association.
D. Reassuring of the child as part of a trusting relationship with an adult.
E. All of the above.

The correct response is option C.

Klein's technique is based on three fundamental principles: play as the child's mode of free association, the existence of transference in children, and the restriction of the analyst's role solely to interpreting unconscious sources of anxiety (Segal 1972). **(p. 975)**

51.2   Although Anna Freud's system of child psychoanalysis was based on the traditional adult model, she recognized that children in analysis differ from adult analysands in which of the following ways?

A. Children do not seek out therapy on their own.
B. Children may have little motivation for cure.
C. Children tend to deny problems and try to externalize their causes rather than accept responsibility for them.
D. Children will run away from discomfort and so will not easily relinquish fantasy for reality.
E. All of the above.

The correct response is option E.

In addition to the above, an additional difference detailed by Freud (1965) is that children prefer the mode of acting to that of talking. **(pp. 976–977)**

51.3   In psychodynamic psychotherapy with children, in contrast to child psychoanalysis,

A. Children are not usually seen 5 days per week.
B. Corrective emotional experiences are encouraged rather than viewed as obstacles to self-awareness.
C. The parents are often greatly involved in treatment.
D. Children are given more active support and practical guidance.
E. All of the above.

The correct response is option E.

All of the above are differences between child psychodynamic psychotherapy and child psychoanalysis. **(p. 977)**

51.4 In regard to how play is conceptualized in psychodynamic psychotherapy, all of the following statements are correct *except*

A. Play is taken as the child's description of his or her perception of the universe.
B. Play is used as a substitute for free association.
C. Children project their inner lives into their play activity.
D. Play is used as a child's mode for communicating the totality of his or her current life.
E. Play allows the child to present his or her predicament "in displacement," as if it did not specifically pertain to the child.

The correct response is option B.

In psychodynamic psychotherapy, play is not used as a substitute for free association, nor is it used for its possible symbolism of unconscious drives or superego sanctions; rather, it is viewed as the child's manner of revealing his or her total life situation. **(p. 978)**

51.5 Evaluating the effectiveness of psychotherapy with children or adolescents is difficult, because a number of factors besides the clinical needs of patients can substantially affect the results. In evaluating study reports of therapeutic effectiveness, which of the following potential influences should be considered?

A. The relative dysfunction of the child's family or environment.
B. The developmental level of the child.
C. The compliance of the parents with therapy recommendations.
D. The extent of treatment goals.
E. All of the above.

The correct response is option E.

Besides the clinical needs of the patient, all of the above factors, as well as the setting of the therapy and the skill of the practitioner, can greatly influence psychotherapy outcomes. **(p. 981)**

References

Freud A: Normality and Pathology in Childhood: Assessments of Development. New York, International Universities Press, 1965

Segal H: Melanie Klein's technique of child analysis, in Handbook of Child Psychoanalysis. Edited by Wolman BB. New York, Van Nostrand Reinhold, 1972, pp 401–414

C H A P T E R   5 2

Cognitive-Behavior Modification

Select the single best response for each question.

52.1   Behavior modification is based largely on two conceptual views of affect, cognition, and behavior: mediational and nonmediational. Which of the following statements describes the *mediational view?*

A. It focuses on direct connections between environmental or situational events and behaviors.
B. It emphasizes constructs such as affect and cognition that underlie behavior.
C. It is the basis for operant conditioning.
D. It conceptualizes child problems as deficits or excesses in performance.
E. None of the above.

The correct response is option B.

The *mediational view* emphasizes constructs such as affect and cognition that mediate or serve as underpinnings of behavior. A critical role is accorded to cognitive process such as plans, goals, beliefs, attributions, and self-statements. The *nonmediational view* focuses on direct connections between environmental or situational events and behavior. Operant conditioning, which views behaviors as a function of prompts or cues, represents a nonmediational view. **(pp. 985–986)**

52.2   Cognitive-behavioral therapy for anxiety in children focuses on dysfunctional cognitions and their implications for the child's subsequent thinking and behavior. The term *cognitive distortions* refers to

A. Attributions that result from cognitive structures, content, and processes.
B. How experiences are processed and interpreted.
C. Information processes that lead to misperceptions of oneself or the environment.
D. Memory and ways in which information is experienced.
E. None of the above.

The correct response is option C.

Cognitive distortions are considered to play a central role in children with anxiety. The term refers to information processes that lead to misperceptions of oneself or the environment. In cognitive-behavioral therapy, four key components of cognition are distinguished: cognitive structures (memory and ways in which information is experienced), cognitive content (ongoing self-statements), cognitive processes (how experiences are processed and interpreted), and cognitive products (attributions that result from cognitive structures, content, and processes). **(p. 990)**

52.3   *Consequential thinking*, an example of a cognitive problem-solving skill, is defined as

A. The ability to identify what might happen as a direct result of acting in a particular way.
B. The ability to relate one event to another over time and to understand why one event led to a particular action.
C. The ability to perceive a problem when it exists and to identify the interpersonal aspects of the confrontation that may emerge.
D. The ability to generate different options that can solve problems.
E. The ability to be aware of the intermediate steps required to achieve a particular goal.

The correct response is option A.

Consequential thinking is the ability to identify what might happen as a direct result of acting in a particular way or choosing a particular solution. *Causal thinking* is the ability to relate one event to another. *Sensitivity to interpersonal problems* is the ability to perceive a problem when it exists. *Alternative-solution thinking* is the ability to generate different options. *Means–end thinking* is the awareness of the intermediate steps required to achieve a goal. **(p. 993, Table 52–2)**

52.4   Parent management training (PMT) is one of the best-researched therapy techniques for children and adolescents. Which of the following statements concerning PMT is *false*?

A. PMT is quite effective in treating conduct disorder.
B. PMT has led to marked improvements in child behavior, as reflected in parent and teacher reports of deviant behavior.
C. Children and adolescents with conduct behavior problems who have been treated with PMT have achieved normative levels of functioning at home and at school.
D. Treatment gains for children treated with PMT are short-lived (less than 6 months).
E. None of the above.

The correct response is option D.

In several studies (e.g., Eyberg et al. 2001), treatment gains from PMT were maintained 1–3 years after treatment, and one group of investigators (Long et al. 1994) reported maintenance of gains 10–14 years after treatment. **(p. 996)**

52.5   Punishment procedures employed in operant conditioning treatments include which of the following?

A. Time-out from reinforcement.
B. Applying response cost.
C. Overcorrection.
D. All of the above.
E. None of the above.

The correct response is option D.

Three punishment methods commonly used with operant conditioning techniques are time-out from reinforcement (removing positive reinforcers for a short time), response cost (removing positive reinforcers such as a token or privilege), and overcorrection (correcting the environmental effects of the inappropriate behavior). **(pp. 998–999)**

References

Eyberg SM, Funderburk BW, Hembree-Kigin TL, et al: Parent-child interaction therapy with behavior problem children: one year maintenance of treatment effects in the family. Child and Family Behavior Therapy 23:1–20, 2001

Long P, Forehand R, Wierson M, et al: Does parent training with young noncompliant children have long-term effects? Behav Res Ther 32:101–107, 1994

C H A P T E R 5 3

Family Therapy

Select the single best response for each question.

53.1 Which of the following is *not* a goal of the psychotherapeutic modality *family therapy?*

A. Exploring the interactional dynamics of the family and their relation to psychopathology.
B. Identifying psychopathology in individual family members and referring them for treatment.
C. Mobilizing the family's internal strengths and functional resources.
D. Restructuring maladaptive interactional family styles.
E. Strengthening the family's problem-solving behavior.

The correct response is option B.

Identifying psychopathology in individual family members and referring them for treatment is not a goal of family therapy. **(p. 1007)**

53.2 Which of the following family therapy investigators developed the concept of the *undifferentiation phenomenon* and its relation to the transmission of anxiety within the family system?

A. Bowen.
B. Bateson.
C. Satir.
D. Minuchin.
E. Haley.

The correct response is option A.

Bowen (1978) pioneered the investigation and observation of family members hospitalized with schizophrenic patients who were related to them. Bateson et al. (1956) and Satir (1967) described communication patterns, cybernetics, systems theory, and the double-bind phenomenon in the early and current life situations of schizophrenic patients. Minuchin (1974) and Haley (1963) established the structural school of family therapy. **(pp. 1008–1009)**

53.3 Different models of family therapy are applicable to different patient populations. Which of the following models is specifically applicable to seriously and chronically disabled families with concomitant disintegration in the family and its social network?

A. Structural and strategic family therapy.
B. Behavioral family therapy.
C. Intergenerational family therapy.
D. Psychodynamic and experiential family therapy.
E. Social network therapy.

The correct response is option E.

Social network therapy is particularly applicable to seriously and chronically disabled families with concomitant disintegration in the family and its social network. **(p. 1010)**

53.4   The theoretical concept of the *boundary* forms the foundation of which of the following types of family therapy?

   A. Contextual therapy.
   B. Experiential family therapy.
   C. Behavioral family therapy.
   D. Structural family therapy.
   E. Psychodynamic family therapy.

   The correct response is option D.

   Structural family therapy, initially developed by Minuchin (1974), has as its foundational theoretical concept the boundary. Clear and flexible boundaries are characteristic of functional families, whereas the members of "enmeshed" or "disengaged" families are, respectively, excessively intrusive or unavailable to one another. **(p. 1011)**

53.5   The rate of relapse among schizophrenic and depressed patients has been reported to be much higher in some families than in others. What family variable has been found to be closely linked to these high relapse rates?

   A. No expressed emotion.
   B. Low expressed emotion.
   C. High expressed emotion.
   D. High cognitive orientation.
   E. Low cognitive orientation.

   The correct response is option C.

   The rate of relapse among schizophrenic and depressed patients in families with high expressed emotion (i.e., negative emotional attitude) is four times higher than that among patients in families with low expressed emotion. **(p. 1022)**

References

Bateson G, Jackson D, Haley J, et al: Toward a theory of schizophrenia. Behav Sci 1:251–264, 1956

Bowen M: Family Theory in Clinical Practice. New York, Jason Aronson, 1978

Haley J: Strategies of Psychotherapy. New York, Grune & Stratton, 1963

Minuchin S: Families and Family Therapy. Cambridge, MA, Harvard University Press, 1974

Satir V: Conjoint Family Therapy. Palo Alto, CA, Science and Behavior Books, 1967

CHAPTER 54

Group Psychotherapy

Select the single best response for each question.

54.1 Which of the following categories of adolescent therapy groups does *not* require a therapeutic contract?

A. Para-analytic psychotherapy groups.
B. Therapeutic groups.
C. Educational and sensitivity groups.
D. Self-help groups.
E. Multifamily groups.

The correct response is option C.

Of the categories above, only the educational and sensitivity group does not require a therapeutic contract. **(p. 1034, Table 54–1)**

54.2 Which of the following statements concerning cognitive-behavior therapy (CBT) groups is *false?*

A. They can be adapted for all age groups.
B. They may be used in a variety of settings.
C. They may be used to treat a variety of presenting problems.
D. They are generally long-term and not skills-specific.
E. In these groups, the child is expected to be an active participant.

The correct response is option D.

CBT groups tend to meet weekly and are generally short-term and often skills-specific. **(p. 1036)**

54.3 Group play therapy

A. Is usually conducted in a large playroom setting.
B. Uses simple and generic play materials.
C. Generally involves weekly meetings.
D. Will vary in length depending on the developmental level of the child.
E. All of the above.

The correct response is option E.

Landreth (1991) suggested choosing toys and materials that encourage creative and emotional expression, engage children, facilitate expressive and exploratory play, allow for expression without verbalization, and permit undirected play. It has been recommended that the age differences of group members not exceed 12 months unless developmental delays are an issue. **(p. 1038)**

54.4 After initial startup tasks, expressive and art therapy group sessions for older children and adolescents consist of four phases. Which of the following is *not* a phase of this modality?

A. Motivation (warm-up).
B. Closure.
C. The art activity.
D. Evaluation of the child's art ability.
E. Discussion of the process and product (sharing).

The correct response is option D.

Evaluation of the child's ability is not part of art therapy groups. Art therapy groups begin by discussing confidentiality and not worrying about the quality of one's product. After this startup, the group session consists of four phases: motivation (warm-up), the art activity itself, discussion of the process and product (sharing), and closure (Chapman and Appleton 1999). **(pp. 1038–1039)**

54.5 Which of the following is a type of self-help group?

A. Permanent group.
B. Addiction group.
C. Crisis group.
D. All of the above.
E. None of the above.

The correct response is option D.

Self-help groups that are useful for patients focus on the individual rather than the diagnosis and can be classified into three categories: crisis, permanent, and addiction groups. **(p. 1040)**

References

Chapman L, Appleton V: Art in group play therapy, in Group Play Therapy: How to Do It, How It Works, and Whom It Is Best For. Edited by Sweeney DS, Homeyer LE. San Francisco, CA, Jossey-Bass, 1999, pp 179–191

Landreth G: Play Therapy: The Art of the Relationship. Muncie, IN, Accelerated Development, 1991, p 116

C H A P T E R   5 5

Hypnosis

Select the single best response for each question.

55.1   An understanding of hypnosis emphasizes the essential features of absorption, dissociation, and suggestibility. *Absorption* is defined as

A. The relative suspension of peripheral awareness.
B. The tendency to accept instruction uncritically.
C. A receptive, trusting rapport.
D. The characteristic state of attentive, receptive focal concentration.
E. None of the above.

The correct response is option D.

Absorption refers to the characteristic state of attentive, receptive focal concentration. *Dissociation* connotes the relative suspension of peripheral awareness that is a by-product of absorption. *Suggestibility* refers to the tendency to accept instruction uncritically, a reflection of the receptive, trusting rapport that is another key feature of hypnosis. **(p. 1043)**

55.2   The Hypnotic Induction Profile (HIP; Spiegel and Spiegel 1978) measures and correlates the subject's patterns of responses to instructions for

A. Eye roll.
B. Dissociation.
C. Posthypnotic arm levitation.
D. Posthypnotic subjective experiences.
E. All of the above.

The correct response is option E.

The HIP measures and correlates the subject's pattern of responses to instructions for eye roll, dissociation, posthypnotic arm levitation, and posthypnotic subjective experiences. **(p. 1045)**

55.3   The greater hypnotizability of children compared with adults is believed to be due to all of the following factors *except*

A. Emotional malleability.
B. Broader cognitive focus.
C. Openness to new experiences.
D. Intrinsic orientation to learning new skills.
E. Ease in accepting regressive phenomena.

The correct response is option B.

Gardner postulated in 1974 that the greater hypnotizability of children was due to their emotional malleability, their general openness to new experiences, their intrinsic orientation to learning new skills, and their greater ease in accepting regressive phenomena. **(p. 1046)**

55.4   Hypnosis has been used to treat a wide array of psychiatric and medical disorders in children and adolescents. Which of the following disorders is the best-established and most systematically studied indication for hypnosis?

   A. Pain.
   B. Seizure disorders.
   C. Anxiety disorders.
   D. Gastrointestinal disorders.
   E. Dissociative identity disorder.

The correct response is option A.

Of the above, pain is the best-established and most systematically studied indication for hypnosis. **(pp. 1046–1048, 1050)**

55.5   Hypnosis is generally *not* appropriate for which of the following mental disorders?

   A. Dissociative identity disorder.
   B. Anxiety disorders.
   C. Childhood habit disorders.
   D. Trichotillomania.
   E. Psychotic disorders.

The correct response is option E.

Hypnosis is generally not appropriate for psychotic disorders. **(pp. 1050–1051)**

References

Gardner G: Hypnosis with children. Int J Clin Exp Hypn 22:20–38, 1974

Spiegel H, Spiegel D: Trance and Treatment: Clinical Uses of Hypnosis. New York, Basic Books, 1978

C H A P T E R   5 6

Milieu Therapy: Inpatient, Partial, Residential

Select the single best response for each question.

56.1   Critical psychological factors for psychiatrists to consider when admitting or discharging children and adolescents who represent a potential danger to themselves or others include the presence of

   A. Persecutory delusions.
   B. Command hallucinations.
   C. Paranoia.
   D. Impaired executive functioning that would take into account the presence of alcohol or substance abuse.
   E. All of the above.

The correct response is option E.

Other psychological factors to consider are the defense mechanisms employed to manage affect, the presence of suspicious vigilance, and the strength of inner control. **(p. 1061)**

56.2   Critical elements of a master treatment plan include all of the following *except*

   A. Psychiatric symptoms.
   B. Insurance coverage.
   C. Medical issues.
   D. Discharge.
   E. Psychoeducation.

The correct response is option B.

Insurance coverage is not a component of master treatment planning. The master treatment plan varies according to the type of program and the population served. Critical elements include psychiatric symptoms, medical issues, education and psychoeducation, and discharge or disposition. **(p. 1061)**

56.3   Which of the following factors differentiates a residential treatment center (RTC) from a psychiatric inpatient unit?

   A. Individuals staying in an RTC perceive themselves as residents rather than as patients.
   B. Meeting of dependency needs is paramount in an RTC.
   C. More regression is expected in an RTC.
   D. All of the above.
   E. None of the above.

The correct response is option A.

An RTC has group living and individual treatment as its focus. Children residing in an RTC perceive themselves as "residents" of the facility rather than as sick persons in a hospital. RTCs expect healthy behavior, rather than the sick behavior that is allowed during a hospital stay. Less regression is expected in an RTC compared with a hospital, where total care and meeting of dependence needs are paramount. **(p. 1063)**

56.4   The focus of inpatient care currently includes all of the following *except*

    A. Transition to less restrictive settings.
    B. Stabilization.
    C. Medical treatment.
    D. Disposition planning.
    E. Assessment.

The correct response is option C.

The focus of inpatient care has become assessment, stabilization, disposition planning, and transition to less restrictive settings. **(p. 1066)**

56.5   Broadly defined, *day treatment* refers to which of the following?

    A. School-based care.
    B. Care provided for at least 5 hours per day.
    C. Integrated education, counseling, and family services.
    D. All of the above.
    E. None of the above.

The correct response is option D.

Day treatment refers to school-based care provided for at least 5 hours a day that involves integrated education, counseling, and family services. By contrast, *partial hospitalization* refers to less than 24-hour care provided in a hospital setting. **(p. 1068)**